Health Status Measurement in Neurological Disorders

Edited by

Crispin Jenkinson

Ray Fitzpatrick

and Damian Jenkinson

RADCLIFFE MEDICAL PRESS

© 2000 Crispin Jenkinson, Ray Fitzpatrick and Damian Jenkinson

Radcliffe Medical Press Ltd
18 Marcham Road, Abingdon, Oxon OX14 1AA

British Library Cataloguing in Publication Data
A catalogue record for this book is available from the British Library.

ISBN 1 85775 399 2

Typeset by Aarontype Ltd, Easton, Bristol
Printed and bound by TJ International Ltd, Padstow, Cornwall

Contents

Preface

The measurement of health from the patient's perspective has become an increasingly central aspect of medical assessment. To date, however, no introductory text on the measurement of patient-based outcomes has been available in neurology. This book highlights the benefits and pitfalls of the application and interpretation of patient-completed measures across a wide range of neurological disabilities. The text aims to give the reader a sense of the breadth of the field as well as its unity. Thus, whilst specific questionnaires have been developed for the different neurological conditions, the methods of development and problems of interpretation are often quite similar. This book will give the reader a critical sense of the benefits of health status measurement in neurology, as well as a working understanding of the issues and concepts. Furthermore, it acts as an introductory guide to what measures are available for use in a variety of neurological disorders. This volume has been produced as a companion guide to *Health Status Measurement: a brief but critical introduction* (1998) (Radcliffe Medical Press, Oxford) which provides a more detailed discussion on the methodologies used in the development and validation of health status measures.

Crispin Jenkinson
Ray Fitzpatrick
Damian Jenkinson
May 2000

List of contributors

Khaled Amar MD, MRCP
Consultant in General Medicine and Geriatric Medicine, Royal Bournemouth and Christchurch Hospitals NHS Trust

Gus A Baker BA, MSc, PhD, FBPsS
Senior Lecturer in Clinical Neuropsychology, Department of Neurosciences, University of Liverpool, Walton Centre for Neurology and Neurosurgery

David Chadwick DM, FRCP
Professor of Neurology, Department of Neurosciences, University of Liverpool, Walton Centre for Neurology and Neurosurgery

Ray Fitzpatrick MA, MSc, PhD, HonMFPHM
Professor of Public Health and Primary Care, Division of Public Health and Primary Health Care, University of Oxford, and Faculty Fellow, Nuffield College, Oxford

Patricia Grey Amante BSc, DipPsych
Senior Researcher, Oxford Outcomes

Alyson Grove MSc
Company Associate, Oxford Outcomes

Jeremy Hobart BSc, PhD, MRCP
Lecturer in Clinical Neurology, Neurological Outcome Measures Unit, Institute of Neurology, London

Ann Jacoby BA, PhD
Professorial Research Fellow in Medical Sociology, Department of Primary Care, University of Liverpool

Crispin Jenkinson BA, MSc, DPhil, HonMFPHM
Deputy Director, Health Services Research Unit, Department of Public Health, University of Oxford

Damian Jenkinson PhD, MRCP
Consultant Physician with special responsibility for Stroke Disease, Royal Bournemouth and Christchurch Hospitals NHS Trust and Clinical Director, Christchurch Hospital

Geir Madland BSc, BDS, FDS, RCS
MRC Clinical Training Fellow, Health Psychology Unit, University College London, and Honorary Registrar in Oral Medicine, Eastman Dental Institute, London

Viv Peto BA
Research Officer, Health Services Research Unit, Department of Public Health, University of Oxford

Tamar Pincus BSc, MSc, MPhil, PhD
Lecturer, Department of Psychology, Royal Holloway, University of London

Paul Quarterman BSc
Partner, Oxford Outcomes

Michael Swash MD, FRCP, FRCPath
Professor of Neurology, St Bartholomew's and the Royal London School of Medicine and Dentistry, Queen Mary and Westfield College, University of London

Alan Thompson MD, FRCP
Professor of Clinical Neurology and Neurorehabilitation, University Department of Clinical Neurology, Institute of Neurology, London

Diane Wild MSc
Partner, Oxford Outcomes

1
Health status measurement in neurology

Crispin Jenkinson, Ray Fitzpatrick and Damian Jenkinson

Introduction

The twentieth century saw an enormous growth in both healthcare provision and research into health and healthcare. Resources and budgets for medical services grew at an exponential rate, as did demand from an expanding population that had ever increasing expectations of healthcare services and a rising elderly population. It seems highly likely, if not inevitable, that the twenty-first century will see demand and expectations continue to develop in the same way. Parallel with this has grown the belief that the systematic evaluation of patients' subjective health status is central to the measurement of illness and disease. Traditionally, evaluation of the patient's perspective did not include their own subjective state, but it is now recognised that clinical evaluation, blood tests and radiological data cannot give a full picture of human health. Measuring health status, or what is sometimes called 'health-related quality of life', is particularly important in those diseases where there is no known cure yet the experience of having the disease can be dramatic. Neurological diseases fall into this category, and present substantial challenges to the measurement of the patient's perspective. Neurology has developed enormously during the past 100 years, and the development of new treatment regimes and pharmaceutical agents must be assessed to determine not only their effect on symptoms and length of life, but also their impact on quality of life. This book provides an introduction to this topic, with particular reference to a number of demanding conditions.

Neurology at the millennium

Over the past century, advances in neurology have triumphed over many infections of the nervous system, using antibiotics and antiviral agents. Enormous improvements in imaging techniques for the nervous system, such as ultrasound, computed tomography and magnetic resonance imaging, have aided diagnosis and treatment. Furthermore, advances in neuroscience, particularly neurophysiology, have resulted in improved diagnostic techniques for identifying disorders of the nervous and neuromuscular systems.[1]

The latter part of the twentieth century saw improved methods of intensive care (e.g. in the management of patients with head injury and stroke), together with great improvement in the techniques of rehabilitation of neurologically impaired individuals. Furthermore, the variety and efficacy of treatment regimes have grown exponentially.

Steven Ringel has argued that neurology was once considered to be a diagnostic specialty without effective treatments. However, he notes that the staggering number of therapeutic options available today has altered this view. Effective management exists for the treatment of migraine, epilepsy, Parkinson's disease and other neurological disorders. The genetic revolution has provided the tools to bioengineer pharmaceuticals that lessen relapses in multiple sclerosis, dissolve a thrombus occluding a cerebral artery, regenerate a damaged peripheral nerve in patients with diabetes, and stimulate stem-cell lines in immuno-suppressed patients. Furthermore, there are now pharmaceuticals that increase survival time in motor neurone disease/amyotrophic lateral sclerosis, and that can improve memory function in Alzheimer's disease. The acceleration of pharmaceutical discoveries is set to continue as knowledge of the molecular and cellular mechanisms of disease increases. This, coupled with the real possibility of gene therapy, means that neurology will be in place to increase not only life expectancy but also quality of life in serious neurological disorders.[2]

Applications of health status measures

A number of potential uses have been suggested for health status measures,[3] but in neurology there are perhaps two central potential areas of application. The most commonly considered applications of health status instruments are as outcome measures in clinical trials or other forms of evaluation. However, it is also argued that they may play as important a role in clinical practice in improving the healthcare of individual patients.

Two related but distinct clinical applications can be identified. They may serve as screening devices, where the primary objective is to identify problems that the health professional might fail to recognise. They may also serve as mechanisms to monitor the course of patients' progress over time, to make decisions about treatment and to assess subsequent therapeutic impact. At present it seems unlikely that health status measures would provide useful screening information in neurology (although questionnaire-based screening tools are commonplace in the related fields of psychiatry and psychology), but they may prove useful in the ongoing evaluation of treatment regimes for patient groups or, indeed, individual patients. In fact, in those instances where there is an absence of biochemical or radiological evidence of health state, neurology has placed considerable value upon clinician-completed instruments to

track disease progression and recovery. For example, the Amyotrophic Lateral Sclerosis (ALS) Functional Rating Scale[4] has been
developed to assess patient change in amyotrophic lateral
sclerosis/motor neurone disease, the Hoehn and Yahr staging score[5] and the Unified Parkinson's Disease Rating Scale[6] are
widely used in Parkinson's disease, and the Barthel Index[7] is
used as a monitoring tool in stroke and head injury patients.[8]
The inclusion of more patient-based assessments may potentially add to clinicians' ability to monitor health status both in
patient groups and potentially in individual cases. However, to
date evidence that such data can influence treatment regimes
and consequent outcomes has been mixed. For example, the
routine feedback of health status data to physicians treating
patients with epilepsy had only a limited impact upon treatment
decisions.[9] Outside the field of neurology, a small number of
studies have begun to examine the impact of use of health status
instruments by clinicians on outcomes, and failed to find
significant benefit. Thus Kazis et al. conducted a trial to examine
the benefits gained by informing clinicians of their patients'
health status scores.[10] The patients all had a diagnosis of rheumatoid arthritis and the health status instrument that was used
varied, being either the Arthritis Impact Measurement Scales or
the Modified Health Assessment Questionnaire. Patients in one
group (the so-called 'experimental group') completed health
status instruments which were sent to clinicians on a quarterly
basis over a year. An 'attention placebo' group completed the
instruments quarterly, but data were not passed on to their
doctor. A control group only completed instruments at the
beginning and end of the study. There were no detectable
differences between groups at the end of the year in process
variables such as changes in medication or referrals to other
agencies. Furthermore, no differences were found in terms of
patient satisfaction or change in health status. A similarly
designed study examined the benefits of using the Functional
Status Questionnaire to screen patients with various disabilities
four times over one year.[11] Again, no differences were found

between the experimental and control groups in either processes of care such as treatment decisions or outcomes in terms of health status. However, such results may indicate that clinicians do not find that the results reported on health status questionnaires are fed back in a meaningful manner, or that the areas in which data are reported are not easily susceptible to clinical manipulation.

Evidence that questionnaire-based data can be useful has been provided by the Dartmouth Primary Care Cooperative Information Project Group (COOP group), who developed a measure for use in primary care. Data on the measure are directly interpretable, and both clinicians and patients have reported favourably on their use as part of the clinical investigation.[12] This highlights the need to make the results obtained from questionnaires readily interpretable. This possibly explains the widespread use of questionnaire-based assessments in psychiatry, where questionnaire scores are directly interpretable (e.g. the Beck Depression Index provides an indication of the level of depression, and the General Health Questionnaire has 'cut-off' points which are taken to indicate the 'caseness' of psychological problems). Measures in neurology and other specialities must be provided with guides to interpretation. Without such information, these questionnaires will simply be providing yet another number, which in itself is not particularly helpful.

The most successful application of health status instruments has been in their use as outcome measures in clinical trials and research evaluations of health interventions. In particular, it is argued that health technologies need to be subjected to randomised controlled trials in which patients are randomly allocated either to receive a treatment that is the subject of investigation or to a control group where they receive either a placebo or a comparable active treatment. This methodology provides the most precise estimate of benefits to patients of an intervention. The wide range of new and developing treatments available in neurology requires assessment with regard to the perceived impact on patient functioning and well-being.

Table 1.1: Criteria by which health assessment questionnaires are evaluated for validity, reliability and responsiveness

Requirements	Definition	Method of assessment
Face validity	Do the questions make sense and do they appear to be relevant for the population from which subjects will be drawn?	Experts in the field and patients with the disease should be asked to read the questions and assess them in terms of ease of comprehension and relevance
Content validity	Is the choice of, and relative importance given to, each question appropriate for the phenomenon being measured?	Experts in the field and patients with the disease should be asked to read the questions and assess them in terms of ease of relevance and, if weighted, they should also determine whether the weights appear to reflect their severity appropriately
Criterion validity	Does the measure produce results that correspond with a superior measure, or does it predict some future criterion value?	Results from one questionnaire may be compared with those of another, but rarely does a 'gold standard' exist, except in cases where the results from a short form of a questionnaire can be compared with the results of an original longer form
Construct validity	Do the results obtained confirm expected relationships or hypotheses?	Results from the questionnaire will be analysed to determine whether it can differentiate between subgroups among which one would expect it to be able to differentiate (e.g. a Parkinson's disease questionnaire would be expected to be able to differentiate between those diagnosed with mild as opposed to severe symptoms)

Requirements	Definition	Method of assessment
Test re-test reliability (reproducibility)	Does the measure produce the same results for different occasions for patients who have experienced no changes?	Results from the questionnaire will be assessed to determine whether they are the same (or very similar) between administrations by, for example, determining that no significant differences exist between the results and that they are highly correlated
Internal consistency reliability	Do the questions in a measure assess the same underlying phenomenon?	A statistical procedure is utilised to determine whether all of the items are highly correlated with each other (the Cronbach's alpha statistic)
Responsiveness	Is the measure sensitive to change?	Statistical procedures are utilised to determine whether a measure is capable of picking up changes in quality of life

Interventions may not always improve quality of life. There are many healthcare interventions which may have a mixture of beneficial and harmful effects on the patient. For example, a wide range of drugs have been developed with beneficial effects of lowering blood pressure, thereby reducing an individual's risk of stroke. At the same time, they may also have negative effects on the patient's mood, social and sexual functioning.[13] Similarly, some patients report adverse effects of pharmaceutical treatment for motor neurone disease. Health status instruments have a vital role to play in providing measures of the extent of harmful effects that may have to be traded off against benefits. Consequently, such measures must be known to have good measurement properties (*see* Table 1.1).[14]

Purpose of this book

The chapters in this book outline the variety of measures that exist for use in neurology, and the ways in which they have been evaluated using established criteria. They document the pros and cons of the instruments available, and provide a brief yet critical introduction to what is currently available. The book covers a wide range of debilitating neurological diseases which have dramatic effects on the day-to-day lives of those who suffer them, and it attempts to provide a guide to how patient experience can be measured meaningfully. The final chapter outlines the requirements for the translation of instruments, given that many of them may be used in cross-cultural treatment trials. It is hoped that this text will stimulate further interest in the field, as well as acting as an introduction to those working in neurology and considering the potential benefits of patient-based assessment.

References

1 Walton J (2000) Clinical neurology. Twentieth century achievements. *Arch Neurol.* **57**: 52.
2 Ringel S (2000) Hey, Mrs Robinson, it's therapeutics! *Arch Neurol.* **57**: 56.
3 Fitzpatrick R (1994) Applications of health status measures. In: C Jenkinson (ed.) *Measuring Health and Medical Outcomes.* UCL Press, London.
4 The ALS CNTF Treatment Study (ACTS) Phase I–II Study Group (1996) The Amyotrophic Lateral Sclerosis Functional Rating Scale. Assessment of activities of daily living in patients with amyotrophic lateral sclerosis. *Arch Neurol.* **53**: 141–7.
5 Hoehn M and Yahr M (1967) Parkinsonism: onset, progression and mortality. *Neurology.* **17**: 427–42.

6   Fahn S and Elton RL (1987) for the UPDRS Development Committee (1987) Unified Parkinson's Disease Rating Scale. In: S Fahn, M Marsden, M Goldstein and DB Calne (eds) *Recent Developments in Parkinson's Disease. Volume 2.* Macmillan, New York.

7   Mahoney FI and Barthel DW (1965) Functional evaluation: the Barthel Index. *Md Med J.* **14**: 61–5.

8   Wade D and Langton Hewer R (1987) Functional abilities after stroke: measurement, natural history and prognosis. *J Neurol Neurosurg Psychiatry.* **50**: 177–82.

9   Wagner AK, Ehrenberg BL, Tran TA *et al.* (1977) Patient-based health status measurement in clinical practice: a study of its impact on epilepsy patients' care. *Qual Life Res.* **6**: 329–41.

10 Kazis LE, Anderson JJ and Meenan RF (1990) Health status as a predictor of mortality in rheumatoid arthritis: a five-year study. *J Rheumatol.* **17**: 609–13.

11 Rubenstein LV, Calkins DR and Young RT (1989) Improving patient function: a randomised trial of functional disability screening. *Ann Intern Med.* **111**: 836–42.

12 Nelson EC, Landgraf JM, Hays RD, Wasson JH and Kirk JW (1990) The functional status of patients: how can it be measured in physicians officers? *Med Care.* **28**: 1111–26.

13 Croog S, Levine S and Testa M (1986) The effects of anti-hypertensive therapy on the quality of life. *N Engl J Med.* **314**: 1657–64.

14 Jenkinson C and McGee H (1998) *Health Status Measurement: a brief but critical introduction.* Radcliffe Medical Press, Oxford.

2
Headache

Tamar Pincus and Geir Madland

Introduction

The aims of this chapter are to provide clinicians and researchers with a comprehensive and critical overview of the instruments used to measure headaches, and an introduction to the theoretical models of pain and measurement in general. The only headache conditions covered are adult migraine and tension-type headache. Physiological measurement is not addressed.

Diagnostic criteria

The measures discussed in this chapter refer to primary (idiopathic) headaches in adults only, comprising migraine and tension-type headache. Cluster headache is not addressed, due to its episodic nature and responsiveness to treatment. Chronic daily headache is excluded because of the lack of consensus on classification.[1]

Migraine is largely considered to be neurochemical, whereas tension-type headache is considered to be purely stress related. However, there is likely to be a complex relationship between stress, mood and migraine,[2] and the aetiology of both conditions is still poorly understood. Moreover, psychophysiological tests, including frontalis electromyography (EMG), temporal blood volume pulse (BVP) and temporal and finger skin temperature, fail to differentiate between the two syndromes.[3]

The difficulties associated with diagnostic criteria are beyond the scope of this chapter and, since chronic headaches are generally considered to be biobehavioural disorders,[4] our review of their measurement is guided by the biopsychosocial model. As yet there is no Cochrane Collaborative Headache Review Group, although this has been called for.[5]

Epidemiology of headaches

Headache is the most common pain syndrome.[4] The lifetime incidence of headache approaches 100%,[6] and nearly three-quarters of the population report recent head pain.[7] The incidence of headache over 12 months in the general adult population is approximately 10% for migraine and 20–30% for frequent (more than monthly) tension-type headache.[8]

The International Headache Society and the ICD-10 guidelines[9] are concerned with pain character (in terms of associated symptoms, such as photophobia), intensity, duration and frequency. Only lip service is paid to psychosocial factors by the inclusion of 'persistent somatoform pain disorder', including 'psychogenic headache', and 'psychological and behavioural factors associated with disorders or diseases classified elsewhere'.

Theories of pain measurement

Models should inform measurements, and although models of pain processing can be complex, the basic international definition of pain clarifies at least some aspects of pain measurement. Pain has been described as 'an unpleasant sensation and emotional experience which is associated with actual or potential tissue damage or is described in terms of such damage'.[10]

Thus pain measurement should primarily consist of of self-report, and should include sensory aspects (e.g. intensity, location and motor implications), affective aspects (e.g. distress and fear),[11] and cognitive aspects (e.g. processing biases[12] and fear avoidance[13]). Some researchers also include behavioural aspects (e.g. function and mobility, pain complaints, etc.).[14] These were often included because patients were not trusted to tell the truth, or because they were unable to describe their pain.[15]

The validity of pain behaviour measurement was tested by Jensen *et al.*, and showed a low correlation with pain intensity.[16] Although 'pain behaviour' is a legitimate topic for research and intervention in its own right, it should not be confused with 'pain experience', which is fundamentally subjective. The same pain behaviour (such as crying) could indicate many different internal states (e.g. fear, suffering or attention-seeking). Pain behaviour, and especially disability, are often conceived of more as the consequences of the pain experience, and also include elements such as general quality of life and well-being, medication consumption and work status. Furthermore, so-called objective measures such as medication consumption are notoriously difficult to measure accurately in headache populations. Two common problems are that individuals are unable or unwilling to report use correctly, and that over-the-counter medications are used far more frequently than prescription medicines, the latter being measurable from prescription redemption and case-files.

There are several reasons for measuring headaches, and there are several aspects of the headache experience that one could measure. Although the measurement should always be as accurate as possible, the depth and breadth of the measurement depend on the primary research question. A global research question (e.g. 'is pharmaceutical A effective in reducing tension headaches when compared to a placebo?') will differ from a clinician's specific query ('has *my* specific intervention helped *this* patient at *this* point in time?'). At the extremes of these two approaches research findings can become meaningless. The attempt to simplify pain measurement and reduce it to a single measure, namely pain intensity, can be misleading. Patients are as concerned with the quality of their pain experience as they are with the intensity, duration and frequency of headaches.[17] However, an attempt to measure every aspect of the patient's life would be unrealistic. The sample needed to provide a statistically significant answer is vast, the analysis itself becomes unworkably complex, and the results are often impossible to interpret.

A tempting solution is to use an instrument or a batch of instruments employed in a previous study published in a well-respected journal. A good outcome study should take into account previous research and apply critical analysis to it. Although it is extremely useful to choose instruments used by other researchers, thus providing the scientific community with an opportunity to carry out a meta-analysis, these instruments may not be appropriate for your patients, their pain experience or their culture. They may be flawed (as will be described later in the chapter), and they may not answer your research question.

The first rule when measuring headaches (or any other pain experience) must therefore be to find out exactly what your research question is, and then (and only then) to choose your design and measurements. Do you want to measure the pain experience *per se* or its consequences?

Reliability and validity

Reliability is a concept that refers to the consistency of the instrument. Typically, in health measurements, researchers focus on test–retest reliability, although internal consistency can be tested in various other ways.[18,19]

Validity, reliability and sensitivity are three concepts that are considered to reflect the quality of an instrument. Validity indicates whether the instrument measures what it is intended to measure, and is often tested against a set criterion, such as another behavioural measurement. If a measurement is found to predict behaviour reliably, it is considered to have good predictive validity. There are many other types of validity, but all of them are basically concerned with interpreting the results obtained from an instrument's scale.[19]

There are at least two points to consider with regard to the validity of measurements in headache. The first is the issue of criterion contamination.[20] Some questionnaires that measure the effect of pain include items about sleep disturbance, lack of appetite and sluggishness. These same items are used to measure depression in other questionnaires.[21] Interpreting high scores on these items becomes difficult. Patients with high scores could be suffering from depression, or they could be particularly affected by their pain experience. Some instruments overcome this problem by adding a specific reference to the pain (e.g. adding 'I have trouble sleeping *because of* my headache'). Although this attribution limits criterion contamination, it is not clear whether such an attribution is shared by patients. If you have great difficulty in sleeping, but you do not attribute it to headaches, do you tick the item? And if not, is the sleep interference not something that clinicians and researchers should know about? In general, questionnaires that use specific attribution to the pain are probably less contaminated and have greater validity than those that do not. One reason for this is that these instruments have been developed specifically for the target population.

Specific measurements in headache

Disease-specific instruments have been demonstrated to be more sensitive to change, have better clinical validity (because they include questions typically asked by clinicians in reference to the pathology) and are more comprehensible to patients.[22] Several headache-specific self-report questionnaires have been developed for research and clinical purposes.

Many researchers simply use a headache index, which is calculated as frequency *multiplied by* intensity.[23–25] Another approach is patient-completed headache forms,[26] which measure the onset, offset, location and intensity of migraine attacks, and any medication taken. These detailed booklets can be easily converted into numerical data, and have been used in randomised controlled trials.[27] Although the information that they provide is clearly useful, they are not considered to measure all aspects of the pain experience. An important advantage of the headache forms is that they can be filled in repeatedly over days or weeks, to give an indication of the course of the patient's headache. This approach is often called a diary method, and is considered to be essential in headache outcome research.[28–30] Typically, measurements are taken four times a day – at breakfast, lunchtime, dinner and bedtime. This also avoids problems with recall.[31]

The Headache Scale[32] is a measure very similar to the McGill Pain Questionnaire (MPQ),[33] but adapted to include adjectives commonly used specifically to describe headaches, rather than pain in general. It includes 30 adjectives, to which patients respond by ticking a 4-point scale, ranging from 0 (= not at all) to 3 (= severely), to indicate the degree to which each adjective describes their pain. The pain descriptors include sensory (pressing, sharp, stabbing) and affective (frightening, distressing, worrying) components, and there is also a 5-point category for severity of the patient's last headache (from 0 = no head-ache to 5 = excruciating headache). The psychometrics of the Headache Scale have not yet been adequately researched, although the test–retest reliability for the total score after one week appears to be lower than the rule-of-thumb criterion of 0.8.[34]

The Headache Disability Inventory (HDI)[35] measures the effect of having headaches on the patient. It consists of a list of 25 statements which are divided into functional and emotional subscales. The functional statements include interference with performing daily tasks, work, social life and achieving goals. The emotional statements include suffering, anger, lack of understanding from others, and confusion. Patients respond to each statement by answering 'yes', 'sometimes' or 'no'. Although the authors report two clear factors, the emotional statements also include a cognitive component (attention distraction, confusion, and inability to think clearly).

The total score and the subscales are significantly related to both headache intensity and frequency, which has been interpreted as evidence for validity. This is not necessarily the case, as the effect of headaches could be independent of severity and frequency. The validity of the questionnaire (i.e. the degree to which it measures what it is claimed to measure) is difficult to assess. In addition to testing the relationship with self-reported pain, information should be gathered on behaviour (e.g. medication consumption, days off work) in relation to functional impact, and on mood (e.g. depression and anxiety) in relation to the emotional impact of headaches. The other psychometric properties reported for this measure are good – 2-month test–retest correlations for the total score and both the sub-scales were above 0.8. An innovative approach to testing validity of a short-term version included a rating of the spouse's perceptions of the patient's perceived assessment of the impact of headaches on their life. Although the correlation fell just short of the criterion of 0.8,[36] this does not necessarily indicate that the questionnaire is invalid. Rather, it probably indicates that many patients suffering from chronic headaches are right when they claim that their spouse does not understand what they are going through! It also suggests that behavioural interventions should include work with the patient and their family.

Measurements of quality of life also exist that are specific to migraines. For example, the 24-hour Migraine Quality-of-Life Questionnaire (24-h MQoLQ)[37] was developed to test the effect of migraine during the immediate 24 hours after onset. The questionnaire includes five domains (work functioning, social functioning, energy, concerns and symptoms) which have been shown to be relatively independent of each other.[38] Construct validity was demonstrated with regard to medication consumption, headache duration, severity and global change in symptoms. The domain subgrouping has proved to be useful in outcome studies.[38] A pharmaceutical vs. placebo study demonstrated a significant difference in three domains (social functioning, symptoms and concerns), but not in the other two (work functioning and energy). The detailed information has clearly appealed to researchers and clinicians. The measure has been translated into 36 languages to date, and is commonly used in clinical trials of migraine.

The Migraine-Specific Quality of Life measure (MSQOL)[39] is a recent measurement that is not yet widely used and includes 25 items on a 4-point Likert scale. In addition, there is a 24-hour diary section designed to measure lost productivity. The items include an evaluation of the long-term effects of migraine (e.g. fear avoidance) as well as purely symptom-based items. It has been found to correlate with scores of frequency of migraines per year, number of symptoms, and number of medical appointments for migraine. The authors propose that it is thereby valid, but regard it as an instrument which measures well-being rather than functional status.

In summary, there are several promising headache-specific quality-of-life measures which may provide sensitive information that cannot be detected by generic instruments. In a comparison with a general quality-of-life instrument (SF-20), the author concludes that the generic instrument may be more useful in defining populations, and the specific instrument in measuring change over time.[40]

The Headache-Specific Locus of Control (HSLC) Scale[41] is a good example of the effect that the biopsychosocial model has had on headache research. The instrument has been adapted from theories of locus of control which categorise individuals' beliefs about control into internal, external (powerful other – healthcare) and external (chance). The psychometric properties of this instrument are reported as satisfactory, although all test–retest correlations fell below 0.8. However, significant relationships were found between scores on the HSLC and symptoms, activity, affect, coping and medication use. This remains a novel and largely untried approach.

Generic measurements

Generic measures of quality of life are increasingly used in all aspects of evaluation in healthcare, and have been used in headache research to assess the wider impact of head pain on self-reported health. The Nottingham Health Profile,[42] Sickness Impact Profile[43] and SF-36[44] have been used in studies of headache and have indicated that the condition can have effects on a wide array of aspects of patients' lives, including not only pain, but also activities of daily living, social functioning, emotional well-being and work behaviour. The Symptoms Checklist (SCL-90),[45] which is a measure of general health, and its shorter version, the Brief Symptom Inventory (BSI),[46] which is a measure of psychological aspects of general health, have been used in headache research, but more to assess risk factors for experiencing head pain than to evaluate the outcome of treatment regimes.[47] These commonly used measures allow for comparisons between headache patients and other groups, facilitate international synthesis of findings, and are considered to be valid and reliable. Generic instruments permit adjustment of raw data for the effects of comorbidity, age and gender on quality of life.[40] In general, it is recommended that outcome studies use a generic quality-of-life instrument as well as measurements that are specific to the target population. The former provide data which can be compared with reference groups and other illness conditions, whilst the latter are likely to measure aspects of ill health that are unique to the patient group under study, and are likely to be more sensitive to changes in health state.

General measures of pain: a brief review

The most popular unidimensional measure of pain intensity is the Visual Analogue Scale (VAS). This is a line, usually 10 cm in length, on which respondents mark the severity of their pain. One end is labelled 'no pain' and the other is labelled 'extreme pain' (or similar descriptors are used), and patients mark their own pain experience between these points. The VAS has many advantages. It is easy to use, fast, requires relatively few instructions, does not depend on language comprehension or education, is easily translated into numerical (and therefore analysable) data, and can be adapted to different times (e.g. pain experienced now, average pain this week). This form of measurement has been shown to have good reliability.[48] Other unidimensional measurements include numerical rating scales (from 0–10 or 1–100), which have been demonstrated to be sensitive to change,[49] are easy to administer and score, and are equally comprehensible across age groups.[16] In combination with a batch of other instruments, these measurements probably yield informative data on one aspect of the pain experience. By themselves, as a measure of headaches, they are inadequate,[49] largely because pain has other attributes in addition to intensity.

A more comprehensive measure of the pain experience is the McGill Pain Questionnaire. The MPQ provides a list of pain descriptors which, when selected by the patient, provide a comprehensive picture of the *quality* of the pain experience, including sensory, affective and evaluative aspects. It also includes a category for intensity. The MPQ has been tested in different cultures, translated into several languages, and used in different patient populations. Its validity and reliability are considered to be high,[48,50] and correlations have been reported between choice of descriptors and diagnosis.[51] However, some of the descriptors appear to be more culture-specific than others (e.g. 'lancinating'). There is a general assumption that the MPQ covers a finite number of pain qualities and, as the descriptors were generated by clinicians, filling in the questionnaire requires a certain standard of education and linguistic mastery.[15] Indeed, one study reported that 15 out of 40 students needed a dictionary to complete the MPQ.[52] Finally, the pain descriptors might not include an essential sensory element specific to the pain experience under investigation (e.g. stiffness, nausea). The MPQ has been used to measure headaches, to compare tension and migraine headaches, and to compare headaches with other pain conditions.[17] Although some concern has been expressed about patients' ability to recall in such detail the quality of a previous pain experience,[53] there is evidence to suggest that headache patients accurately recall the quality of the pain up to one week later.[54]

The West Haven Yale Multidimensional Pain Inventory (WHYMPI or MPI)[55] is a detailed multi-dimensional instrument. Three of the 12 subscales measure the impact of pain on patients' lives, the response of others to patients' pain, and interference with daily activities. The instrument has been shown to be sensitive to change, reasonably reliable and valid. Some of the subscales, especially the one that measures pain interference, appear to have great meaning for patients. Three clusters of patients are consistently identified, namely 'dysfunctional', 'interpersonally distressed' and 'adaptive copers'.[15,56] In a study of validity of the MPI, headache patients could not be differentiated from patients in the other pain groups, but the results indicated that the MPI is a valid measure of the cognitive, behavioural and affective aspects of pain.[56] It was suggested that treatment might be tailored to each patient cluster.

The Illness Perception Questionnaire (IPQ)[57] and the Coping Strategies Questionnaire (CSQ)[58] have also been used to assess headache patients' cognitions. They indicate that primary headache is considered severe and debilitating relative, for example, to temporomandibular joint pain, that psychological distress appears to be provoked by pain and stress, and that passive coping strategies and perceptions contribute to that distress.[59]

Novel measurements: a patient-based approach

One way to choose an outcome measure is to look not at what is measurable but at what is important – and at what is important to *patients*. This approach is described as patient based, and is finding some support among clinicians and healthcare researchers. An example of this approach is the Measure Yourself Medical Outcome Profile (MYMOP).[60] This innovative approach to measuring outcome in primary care has concentrated specifically on the aspects and the effects of the illness which the patient decides are most important. This increases the sensitivity to within-person change over time, thus satisfying clinical needs, whilst also providing a brief and simple instrument that yields numerical data. Patients select two (or more) symptoms which they most want changed, and they indicate how severe these have been over the previous week. They then select one activity they cannot currently engage in, and give a score for their general sense of well-being. The psychometric properties reported in the original research appear promising, and the instrument has the advantage of easy and valid adaptation to different disorders.

Good practice: measuring adverse effects

A common mistake in outcome research is the failure to assess adverse effects. Diaries in the measurement of headaches are well suited to the provision of information on adverse effects. These should include differences between treatment and placebo, frequency and type, and explicit statements that no adverse effects occurred. These adverse effects should also be weighted according to their importance to patients. This information can be translated into an intuitively comprehensible numerical value, such as numbers needed to harm (NNH), provided that research has clarified what adverse effects patients are willing or unwilling to endure.

Good practice: time lines

Once the research question has been clarified, the variable to be tested will become apparent, and a reliable and valid instrument can be selected. However, it will still be necessary to consider when and how often to measure. Time lines (the frequency with which change occurs) are particularly difficult to establish in headache, and instead of looking at one end-point (e.g. 'headache present or absent after 48 hours'), it may be preferable to look at a pattern. This can be difficult to analyse (repeated-measures analysis is notoriously complex), but it is better practice to search for a statistical analysis that will answer the research question than to change the research question to fit the analysis.

Conclusion and summary

The measurement of headaches and of the interaction between the headache experience and the patient's well-being should be informed by models of pain and theories of measurement. Consideration should be given to clarifying the research question before an instrument is selected. There is now a choice between reliable and valid instruments specific to headache, and widely used generic instruments. There are pros and cons influencing the choice of either of these. Finally, new patient-focused approaches are being developed, and these may yield information that is relevant not only to those investigating and intervening, but also to those who experience the headaches at first hand.

References

1 Silberstein SD and Lipton RB (1997) Chronic daily headache. In: PJ Goadsby and SD Silberstein (eds) *Headache*. Butterworth Heinemann, Oxford.

2 Spierings E, Sorbi M, Maassen G and Honkoop P (1997) Psychophysical precedents of migraine in relation to the time of onset of the headache: the migraine time line. *Headache.* **37**: 217–20.

3 Lichstein K, Fischer S, Eakin T, Amberson J, Bertorini T and Hoon P (1991) Psychophysiological parameters of migraine and muscle-contraction headaches. *Headache.* **31**: 27–34.

4 Schoenen J and Maertens de Noordhout A (1994) Headache. In: PD Wall and R Melzack (eds) *Textbook of Pain* (3e). Churchill Livingstone, Edinburgh.

5 Steiner TJ (1998) Treating headache from an evidence base: the Cochrane Collaboration. *Cephalalgia.* **18 (Supplement 21)**: S63–5.

6 Ho K-H, Ong B and Lee S-C (1997) Headache and self-assessed depression scores in Singapore University undergraduates. *Headache.* **37**: 26–30.

7 Koutantji M, Pearce S and Oakley D (1998) The relationship between gender and family history of pain with current pain experience and awareness of pain in others. *Pain.* **77**: 25–31.

8 Rasmussen BK and Olesen J (1994) Epidemiology of migraine and tension-type headache. *Curr Opin Neurol.* **7**: 264–71.

9 International Headache Classification Committee (1997) *ICD-10 Guide for Headaches.* World Health Organisation, Geneva.

10 Merskey H, Albe-Fessard DG, Bonica JJ *et al.* (1979) International Association for the Study of Pain Sub-Committee on Taxonomy. *Pain.* **6**: 249–52.

11 Leventhal H and Everhart D (1979) Emotion, pain and physical illness. In: CA Izard (ed.) *Emotions in Personality and Psychopathology.* Plenum Press, London.

12 Pincus T, Pearce S, McClelland A and Isenberg D (1995) Endorsement and memory bias for pain stimuli in pain patients. *Bri J Clin Psychol.* **34**: 267–77.

13 Vlaeyen JW, Seelen HA, Peters M, de-Jong P, Aretz E, Beisiegel E and Weber W (1999) Fear of movement/(re)injury and muscular reactivity in chronic low back pain patients: an experimental investigation. *Pain.* **82**: 297–304.

14 Fordyce WE (1983) The validity of pain behaviour measurement. In: R Melzack (ed.) *Pain Measurement and Assessment.* Raven Press, New York.

15 Skevington SM (1995) *Psychology of Pain.* John Wiley & Sons, Chichester.

16 Jensen M, Karoly P and Braver S (1986) The measurement of clinical pain intensity: a comparison of six methods. *Pain.* **27**: 117–26.

17 Philips HC (1983) Chronic headache experience. In: R Melzack (ed.) *Pain Measurement and Assessment.* Raven Press, New York.

18 Elmes DG, Kantowitz BH and Roediger HL III (1995) *Research Methods in Psychology.* West Publishing Company, St Paul, MN.

19 Bowling A (1997) *Measuring Health* (2e). Open University Press, Buckingham.

20 Pincus T, Callaghan LF, Bradley LA, Vaughn WK and Wolfe F (1986) Elevated MMPI scores for hypochondriasis, depression and hysteria in patients with rheumatoid arthritis reflect disease rather than psychological status. *Arthritis Rheumatol.* **29**: 1456–66.

21 Beck A, Ward C, Mendelson M, Mock J and Erbaugh J (1961) An inventory for measuring depression. *Arch Gen Psychiatry.* **4**: 561–71.

22 Ruta D, Garratt A, Wadlaw D and Russell I (1994) Developing a valid and reliable measure of health outcome for patients with low back pain. *Spine.* **19**: 1887–96.

23 Sartory G, Muller B, Metsch J and Pothmann R (1998) A comparison of psychological and pharmacological treatment of pediatric migraine. *Behav Res Ther.* **36**: 1155–70.

24 Mitsikostas DD, Gatzonis S, Thomas A and Ilias A (1997) Buspirone vs. amitriptyline in the treatment of chronic tension-type headache. *Acta Neurol Scand.* **96**: 247–51.

25 Pini LA, Bigarelli M, Vitale G and Sternieri E (1996) Headaches associated with chronic use of analgesics. *Headache.* **36**: 433–9.

26 Bakal DA and Kaganov JA (1976) A simple method for self-observation of headache frequency, intensity and location. *Headache.* **16**: 123–4.

27 Thomas M, Behari M and Ahuja GK (1991) Flunarizine in migraine prophylaxis: an Indian trial. *Headache.* **31**: 613–15.

28 de Bruijn-Kofman AT, van de Wiel H, Groenman NH, Sorbi MJ and Klip E (1996) Effects of a mass-media behavioral treatment for chronic headache: a pilot study. *Headache.* **37**: 415–20.

29 Blanchard EB, Appelbaum KA, Nicholson NL *et al.* (1991) A controlled evaluation of the addition of cognitive therapy to a home-based biofeedback and relaxation treatment of vascular headache. *Headache.* **30**: 371–6.

30 Andrasik F (1992) Assessment of patients with headaches. In: D Turk and R Melzack (eds) *Handbook of Pain Assessment.* Guildford Press, New York.

31 Epstein L and Abel G (1977) An analysis of biofeedback training effects for tension headache headache patients. *Behav Ther.* **8**: 37–47.

32 Hunter M (1983) The Headache Scale: a new approach to the assessment of headache pain based on pain descriptions. *Pain.* **16**: 361–73.

33 Melzack R (1975) The McGill Pain Questionnaire: major properties and scoring method. *Pain.* **1**: 277–99.

34 Jahanshahi M, Hunter M and Philips C (1986) The Headache Scale: an examination of its reliability and validity. *Headache.* **26**: 76–82.

35 Jacobson G, Ramadan N, Aggarwal S and Newman C (1994) The Henry Ford Hospital Headache Disability Inventory (HDI). *Neurology.* **44**: 837–42.

36 Jacobson G, Ramadan N and Norris L (1995) The Headache Disability Inventory (HDI): short-term test–retest reliability and spouse perceptions. *Headache.* **35**: 534–9.

37 Hartmaier S, Santanello N, Epstein N and Silberstein S (1995) Development of a brief 24-hour migraine-specific quality-of-life questionnaire. *Headache.* **35**: 320–9.

38 Santanello N, Hartmaier S, Epstein R and Silberstein S (1995) Validation of a new quality-of-life questionnaire for acute migraine headache. *Headache.* **35**: 330–7.

39 Wagner TH, Patrick DL, Galer BS and Berzon RA (1996) A new instrument to assess the long-term quality-of-life effects from migraine: development and psychometric testing of the MSQOL. *Headache.* **36**: 484–92.

40 Solomon GD (1997) Evolution of the measurement of quality of life in migraine. *Neurology.* **48 (Supplement 3)**: S10–15.

41 Martin NJ, Kenneth MS, Holroyd A and Penzien DB (1990) The Headache-Specific Locus of Control scale: adaptation to recurrent headaches. *Headache.* **30**: 729–34.

42 Passchier J, Mourik J, Brienen JA and Hunfeld JAM (1998) Cognitions, emotions, and behavior of patients with migraine when taking medication during an attack. *Headache.* **38**: 458–64.

43 Carlsson J, Augustinsson L-A, Blomstrand C and Sullivan M (1990) Health status in patients with tension headache treated with acupuncture or physiotherapy. *Headache.* **30**: 593–9.

44 Litaker DG, Solomon GD and Genzen JR (1997) Using pretreatment quality-of-life perceptions to predict response to sumatriptan in migraineurs. *Headache.* **37**: 630–4.

45 ter Kuile MM, Spinhoven P, Linssen ACG and van Houwelingen HC (1995) Cognitive coping and appraisal processes in the treatment of chronic headaches. *Pain.* **64**: 257–64.

46 Derogatis LR (1979) *Brief Symptom Inventory.* Clinical Research, Baltimore, MD.

47 Gilbar O, Bazack Y and Harel Y (1997) Gender, primary headache and psychological distress. *Headache.* **38**: 31–4.

48 McQuay H (1990) Assessment of pain and effectiveness of treatment. In: D Costain and A Hopkins (eds) *Measuring the Outcomes of Medical Care.* Royal College of Physicians, London.

49 Lee V and Rowlingson J (1996) Defining quality of life in chronic pain. In: B Spilker (ed.) *Quality of Life and Pharmacoeconomics in Clinical Trials.* Lippincott-Raven, Philadelphia, PA.

50 Bradley A (1993) Pain measurement in arthritis. *Arthritis Care Res.* **6**: 178–86.

51 Reading AE, Hand DJ and Sledmere CM (1983) A comparison of response profiles obtained on the McGill Pain Questionnaire and an adjective checklist. *Pain.* **16**: 375–83.

52 Klepac RK, Dowling J, Rokke P, Dodge L and Schafer L (1981) Interview vs. pencil and paper administration of the McGill Pain Questionnaire. *Pain.* **11**: 241–6.

53 Jones E (1997) Pain. *Int J Psychoanal.* **38**: 255.

54 Hunter M, Philips C and Rachman S (1979) Memory for pain. *Pain.* **6**: 35–46.

55 Kerns RD, Turk DC and Rudy TE (1985) The West Haven – Yale Multidimensional Pain Inventory (WHYMPI). *Pain.* **23**: 345–56.

56 Walter L and Brannon L (1991) A cluster analysis of the Multidimensional Pain Inventory. *Headache.* **31**: 476–9.

57 Weinman J, Petrie KJ, Moss-Morris R and Horne R (1996) The Illness Perception Questionnaire: a new method for assessing the cognitive representation of illness. *Psychol Health.* **11**: 431–45.

58 Rosenstiel A and Keefe F (1983) The use of coping strategies in chronic low back pain patients: relationship to patient characteristics and current adjustment. *Pain.* **17**: 33–44.

59 Madland G, Feinmann C and Newman S (1999) Cognitions, behaviours, distress and pain in temporomandibular

disorder and primary headache. Presentation to the Annual Conference of the Division of Health Psychology of the British Psychological Society, Leeds, 1–3 September 1999.

60 Paterson C (1996) Measuring outcomes in primary care: a patient-generated measure, MYMOP, compared with the SF-36 health survey. *BMJ.* **312**: 1016–21.

3
Parkinson's disease

Viv Peto, Crispin Jenkinson and Ray Fitzpatrick

Introduction

Parkinson's disease (PD) is a common, chronic neurological condition affecting just over 1 in 1000 people and increasing in incidence in older age groups.[1] Early diagnosis is difficult, but is usually defined by the presence of at least two of the primary physical symptoms (tremor, rigidity, bradykinesia and postural instability), as well as a positive response to the drug levodopa. These primary symptoms can manifest themselves in many ways, including slowness, stiffness and the inability to initiate movement, a stooped posture, an impassive face and a shuffling gait. There may be difficulties with walking and balance, dressing, speech and communication, loss of dexterity, or fatigue. As the disease progresses, the physical symptoms may affect other aspects of daily life and create additional psychological and social problems. Currently there is no cure for PD, although treatment can be very effective, at least in the early stages, in managing some of the symptoms, and in extending life expectancy. However, in the long term the primary aim of any treatment must be to improve quality of life.

Until recently, the impact of PD on patients' lives had largely been assessed by clinical scales such as the Hoehn and Yahr Scale,[2] the Columbia Rating Scale[3] and the Unified Parkinson's

Disease Rating Scale (UPDRS),[4] the latter incorporating a modified Hoehn and Yahr Scale, rated in eight stages, and also measuring activities of daily living, as assessed by the clinician, by incorporating the Schwab and England scale.[5] These measures focus mainly on neurological symptoms and physical impairment (indeed, the Schwab and England scale is a more accurate measure of physical independence than of activities of daily living). Thus, for example, evidence of effectiveness in relation to disability of a drug such as Selegiline has tended to come largely from such clinical scales,[6] and by assessment of the primary symptoms of the disease, notably tremor, rigidity, bradykinesia (i.e. abnormally slow body movements) and postural instability.

However, within the neurological community there is growing interest in measuring health status from the patient's perspective. This chapter outlines the increasing use of health-related quality-of-life measures in the field of Parkinson's disease. Such measures are intended to assess a broader range of areas of the patient's well-being than is assessed by clinical scales.

Important areas of health-related quality of life in PD

Although there is no consensus on the definition of health-related quality of life in medical research, there is nevertheless broad agreement that the focus should be on areas of experience of greatest concern to individuals who have the relevant health problem, and that the concept of health-related quality of life is multi-dimensional.[7,8] Research has indicated some of the important concerns for individuals with PD. Bulpitt et al.[9] have shown that some symptoms, such as being frozen to the spot, grimacing, and jerking of the arms and legs, are between 20 and 40 times more frequently experienced by individuals with PD than by other individuals of the same age, whilst a diverse range of other experiences, such as loss of interest in sex, and indigestion and headache, are very commonly experienced by individuals with PD, although there is disagreement about the extent to which these problems exceed those of age-matched controls.[10] Sleep-related problems are frequently reported, inability to turn over in bed and nocturnal cramps being reported by more than 50% of one sample of individuals with PD.[11]

Several epidemiological surveys have demonstrated the importance of physical disability in PD, particularly in relation to walking, moving around in bed and in the house, and mobility in public areas.[1,12] Falls are a common hazard for individuals with PD, and in one study 13% of patients reported falls occurring more than once a week.[13] As a result, hip fractures can be a common health problem in this group of patients. Individuals with PD report more work-related problems than matched controls, and they also report more limitations with regard to household management.[14] The potential social consequences of PD are diverse. Individuals may experience social isolation and limited leisure activities; in one study 50% of individuals with PD compared to 27% of age-matched controls reported restricted social activities.[15] Over two-thirds of individuals attending a specialist clinic for PD reported giving up a hobby because of their PD.[16] The same series of patients commonly reported difficulties in taking holidays. Within the household, individuals with PD rate their home or family life as being far more adversely affected by health problems than do controls.

Financial difficulties may be an important consequence of PD. Oxtoby estimated that 19% of individuals with PD experienced such problems.[17] Premature retirement from work, resulting in reduced income, was reported by 29% of individuals with PD in a study of quality of life of patients with PD attending a specialist clinic. Rubenstein et al. reported a case–control study of individuals with PD identified from the US population-based National Medical Expenditure Survey.[18] Individuals with PD faced significantly more health-related economic costs than did matched controls, due to costs of prescriptions, home care and hospitalisation. They were also significantly more likely to report that their health prevented them from working or limited the kind of paid work that they could do.

Emotional well-being is a central aspect of health-related quality of life. Up to 30% of individuals with PD experience depression.[19,20] Less severe but nevertheless important effects include a sense of loss of control over one's life, loss of confidence, embarrassment and stigma arising from the symptoms of PD.[21] The consequences of cognitive impairment are also distressing. Bulpitt *et al.* found that 33% of individuals were concerned about problems of concentration.[9] Severe cognitive decline and dementia give rise to further stresses. PD can involve specific problems with communication, and approximately one-third of individuals with PD experience speech difficulties that cause them concern.[1,12]

Health status measures

Measures of health-related quality of life (hereafter termed 'health status measures', for the sake of brevity) are intended to assess salient aspects of disease from the patient's perspective in a way that produces standardised and valid information. It is equally important that such information is collected in a feasible and acceptable manner, so that data collection in clinical trials does not jeopardise the care of participating patients.

There are two main types of health status measure that have been developed for use in clinical trials, namely generic and disease-specific measures. Both types have been used in relation to PD, but the two types differ in their form, content and intended purpose.

Generic measures

Generic measures, as implied by the name, are intended to be relevant to a wide spectrum of health problems, rather than to a single specific disease. The main advantage of such an instrument is that it allows comparisons of health status across diverse patient groups. They tend to be worded in such a way that questionnaire items are relevant to the vast majority of a community. This has the advantage that estimates of the health status of a population as a whole can be made as a baseline or norm against which to evaluate the scores of a specific patient group or intervention. Three of the most widely used generic measures are the Sickness Impact Profile (SIP),[22] (anglicised for use in the UK as the Functional Limitations Profile[23]), the Nottingham Health Profile (NHP)[24] and the 36-Item Short-Form Health Survey (SF-36)[25] (see Box 3.1).

There is now reasonable evidence of the use of such generic measures in PD. The SIP was administered by Longstreth et al. to patients with PD attending a neurological clinic, and to matched controls.[15] SIP scale scores correlated significantly with Hoehn and Yahr and Columbia scale scores assessed by the neurologist, providing evidence of construct validity. The correlations with the clinical scales were somewhat stronger for physical than for psychosocial dimensions of the SIP, and the investigators concluded that the SIP assesses important effects of PD that are not detected by the conventional neurological scales. The problem most commonly reported by patients (75% of cases) was difficulty in writing. The areas that showed the greatest difference from controls included various items regarding housework, sexual interest, problems of speech and social activities, in all of which patients with PD had poorer scores. Another study used the SIP to demonstrate greater problems for individuals with PD in relation to physical function than were observed in a general population survey of individuals identified as disabled.[14] Finally, dimensions of the SIP have been found to be sensitive to change, and to be able to differentiate between standard carbidopa-levodopa and sustained-release carbidopa-levodopa.[26]

The NHP has also been used to demonstrate higher levels of problems across all six dimensions for individuals with PD compared to a control group of the same age.[27] Similarly, the

---

Box 3.1: Features of the SIP/FLP, NHP and SF-36

Sickness Impact Profile (SIP)/Functional Limitations Profile (FLP)
12 dimensions: 136 items
- Ambulation
- Household management
- Emotion
- Eating
- Body care and movement
- Recreation and pastimes

- Alertness
- Communication
- Mobility
- Social interaction
- Sleep and rest
- Work

Other
- The FLP is the anglicised version of the SIP
- An overall single index score can be derived from the FLP/SIP, as can a psychosocial dimension score and a physical dimension score

Nottingham Health Profile (NHP)
6 dimensions: 38 items
- Energy
- Sleep

- Pain
- Social isolation

- Emotional reactions
- Physical mobility

Other
- A single index (NHP distress index) can be created from a subset of the items

Short-Form 36-Item Health Survey (SF-36)
8 dimensions: 36 items
- Physical functioning
- Social functioning
- Pain
- Energy
- Mental health

- Health perception
- Role limitations due to physical problems
- Role limitations due to emotional problems

Other
- Two summary scores can be derived from the SF-36, namely the physical component summary (PCS) and the mental component summary (MCS)

---

membership of PD societies reported poorer scores on all dimensions of the SF-36 than did controls.[28]

The SF-36 has been found to provide consistent strong associations between Hoehn and Yahr stage and SF-36 dimensions.[29] Furthermore, the mental health dimension of the SF-36 has been found to be responsive to intervention. Mercer reports the use of a simple subset of items taken from the SF-36 to evaluate the impact of a health management programme, 'PROPATH', on the well-being of patients with PD.[30] The PROPATH programme is intended to provide advice and information to help patients to cope with the physical and psychosocial consequences of PD. Although there was no apparent impact on patient satisfaction measures, a significant improvement was detected in the five-item measure of mental health (the mental health dimension of the SF-36) one year after the intervention.

Some criticisms of the use of generic measures have been raised, notably that the SIP is too long a questionnaire to be useful in all situations where quality-of-life measures might profitably be included, the NHP is insensitive to lower levels of ill health, and the terminology of the SF-36 renders it unsuitable for older adults, as many of the questions ask about work-related behaviour.[31] However, despite such concerns, the measures appear to be reliable and to provide a meaningful and useful insight into the demands of the illness on patients who are affected by it.

Generic measures of quality of life are not designed for a particular disease, and consequently they have some limitations. For example, although they include questions about physical, social or psychological factors, they often omit questions that are specifically relevant to particular disease groups, such as issues concerning the social embarrassment which individuals with PD may experience. Thus a PD-specific questionnaire is intended to give a more accurate picture of the impact of PD than a generic measure. It is also more likely to be able to detect the small but important changes that are anticipated with many of the modern drug therapies.

There are three disease-specific measures of quality of life in PD, namely the Parkinson's Impact Scale (PIMS),[32] the Parkinson's Disease Quality-of-Life Questionnaire (PDQL)[33] and the

---

Box 3.2: Features of the PDQL and PDQ-39

Parkinson's Disease Quality-of-Life Scale (PDQL)
4 dimensions: 37 items
- Parkinsonian symptoms
- Systemic symptoms
- Emotional functioning
- Social functioning

Parkinson's Disease Questionnaire (PDQ-39)
8 dimensions: 39 items
- Mobility
- Activities of daily living
- Emotional well-being
- Bodily discomfort
- Stigma
- Social support
- Cognition
- Communication

Associated measures
- PDQ-39SI: single index derived from the PDQ-39
- PDQ-8SI: single index derived from the PDQ-8
- PDQ-8: an 8-item measure containing the most highly correlated item from each PDQ-39 dimension, designed solely to provide the PDQ-8SI

39-item Parkinson's Disease Questionnaire (PDQ-39).[34,35] The PIMS was designed on the basis of clinical judgement whereas the PDQL and PDQ-39 were based on patient interviews. The dimensions of the PDQL and PDQ-39 are shown in Box 3.2.

The Parkinson's Impact Scale (PIMS)

The PIMS is a short measure that was developed on the basis of clinical judgement, with its 10 items designed by nurses from PD specialty clinics. Data collected by the developers of the PIMS on 149 PD patients suggest that this measure has acceptable levels of reliability and validity. Because of its brevity, Calne *et al.* suggest that the PIMS is of potential use in clinical settings, and may be applicable to other chronic illnesses.[32]

However, health status measures should ideally be based on patient reports rather than clinical judgements. Consequently, we shall describe the PDQL and PDQ-39 in greater detail. Both of these measures have been developed according to widely accepted criteria for the construction of disease-specific quality-of-life measures.[36] The criteria are that questions included in the measure should reflect areas of quality of life that are important to the specific patient group under study, and that they should measure aspects of physical, social and psychological well-being. In addition, the scores generated from the measure should be amenable to statistical analysis, the questionnaire should fulfil tests for validity, and it should be as short as possible and simple to complete. A review of health status quality-of-life measures found that both the PDQL and the PDQ-39 fulfilled most of these criteria.[37]

The Parkinson's Disease Quality-of-Life Questionnaire (PDQL)

The PDQL was developed in two phases. In the first phase, potential questions for a questionnaire were generated by a combination of in-depth interviews with four patients, and suggestions from neurologists, members of the Dutch PD Society and a literature review. Then 13 patients were asked to rate the relative importance of 73 candidate questionnaire items, the result of this task being the generation of a list of the 37 most important items. In the second phase, the completed answers to the PDQL of 384 members of the Dutch PD Society were analysed in conjunction with demographic variables and answers to other quality-of-life measures. The answers from the larger survey were factor-analysed to produce the four scales of the PDQL. Furthermore, the PDQL had expected patterns of correlation with the other quality-of-life measures. The developers have made several important observations that are relevant to any assessment of quality of life in this group of patients. First, they note that patients with PD take twice as long to complete a questionnaire as a comparison group of patients with inflammatory bowel disease. This highlights the advantages of brevity and simplicity when assessing quality of life in patients with PD. Secondly, the developers note that individuals with substantial cognitive impairment will have problems completing such assessments. Although they estimate that only 1% of their sample showed such impairment, this may be a greater problem in other studies, and it could result in bias in trials if non-response is not taken into consideration.

In assessment of the PDQL on a PD sample derived from a community-based register, Hobson *et al.* found it to be a valid instrument which could be an important additional measure reflecting the impact of PD from the patient's perspective.[38] However, they reported that the responsiveness of this measure has yet to be determined.

The Parkinson's Disease Questionnaire (PDQ-39)

To ensure that the questionnaire captured aspects of health status that are important to patients, in-depth interviews were conducted with 20 individuals with PD attending a neurology out-patient clinic. Patients were asked to describe those areas of their lives which had been adversely affected by PD. This generated a large number of possible questionnaire items which could be included in the final questionnaire. These items were scrutinised for ambiguity and repetition. A 65-item question-naire was then developed and piloted to test its basic accept-ability and comprehension.

The next stage was to reduce the number of questionnaire items and to generate scales for the different dimensions of health-related quality of life. A total of 359 individuals completed the 65-item questionnaire. Factor analyses produced a 39-item questionnaire with eight dimensions. Reliability in terms of the internal consistency of each dimension was assessed using the Cronbach's alpha statistic,[39] where values of >0.5 are acceptable, although ideally scores should be >0.7.[40,41] Internal consistency was found to be good for all dimensions of the PDQ-39, and comparable to other established health status measures.[28] The result was the PDQ-39, a questionnaire with 39 items covering eight discrete dimensions (*see* Box 3.2). The scores from each dimension are computed into a scale ranging from 0 (best, i.e. no problem at all) to 100 (worst, i.e. maximum severity of problem).

The measurement properties of the PDQ-39, its reliability, validity and sensitivity to change, were assessed using data from a second postal survey and an out-patient clinic sample.[42] For the second postal survey, all members with PD from five different PD Society branches were posted a booklet containing the PDQ-39, a generic health status measure (the SF-36) and questions about the severity of their PD symptoms. In addition, a second copy of the PDQ-39 was included in a sealed envelope. Respondents were asked to complete the second copy 3 to 6 days after the first, and were asked to report any important changes in their health during that time.

In the clinic sample, individuals with PD attending neurology out-patient departments were surveyed with the PDQ-39 and the SF-36 and clinically assessed using the Hoehn and Yahr Index and the Columbia Rating Scale, and were reassessed using the same measures 4 months later.

Reliability

The two sets of PDQ-39 data from the second postal survey were available to examine the reliability in terms of internal consistency of the eight PDQ-39 dimensions. Cronbach's alpha was satisfactory for all scales on both occasions, with the exception of social support (0.66) at time 1, which was only slightly below the accepted criterion. The test–retest reliability (reproducibility) was examined by means of correlation co-efficients between scale scores at time 1 and time 2. The correlations were all significant ($P < 0.001$), and a *t*-test for changes in the distribution of scores between the two assessments produced no significant differences ($P < 0.05$).

Validity

Construct validity was examined by means of correlations of scale scores with relevant SF-36 scores. The correlations of PDQ-39 scales with matching scales of SF-36 were all significant. Questionnaire items asked respondents to assess the severity of their tremor, stiffness and slowness. A consistent pattern of poorer scores on all PDQ-39 scales was obtained for patients with more severe self-assessed symptoms. Further evidence of construct validity has been established in a Spanish study which compared the Unified Parkinson's Disease Rating Scale (UPDRS) with the PDQ-39. All of the PDQ-39 scales were significantly correlated with the UPDRS score.[43]

The validity of the PDQ-39 was also examined with regard to agreement with clinical assessments performed by the neurologists in the clinic study (the Hoehn and Yahr Index and the Columbia Rating Scale). Significant correlations were found between both clinical scales and the PDQ-39 dimensions ($P < 0.05$) for all dimensions except social support.

Sensitivity to change

Sensitivity to change of a quality-of-life instrument is particularly important in view of potential applications in clinical trials. This was tested on data from the clinic sample to determine whether changes in PDQ-39 scores over a 4-month period were consistent with patients' global retrospective judgements of change. Changes in PDQ-39 scores were calculated as standardised response means (the change in score for a measure divided by the standard deviation of that change in score). Changes for two dimensions of the PDQ-39, namely mobility and activities of daily living (ADL), were significant ($P < 0.01$; paired t-test), and standardised response means (SRMs) suggested moderate deterioration (0.55 and 0.43, respectively) for the sample that described themselves as worse in their global retrospective judgements after 4 months. According to conventional criteria,[44] SRMs of this magnitude indicate moderate levels of change, which suggests reasonable responsiveness for these two dimensions. For all of the patients, their retrospective judgement of change correlated significantly with the change in scores for mobility and ADL. The change in scores was examined in relation to patterns of change in the SF-36 physical and mental summary scores,[45] and the correlations were significant for five PDQ-39 scales (mobility, ADL, emotional well-being, stigma and social support). There is therefore some evidence of sensitivity to change in some dimensions of the PDQ-39 which are not detected by conventional clinical measures.

Discussion and conclusion

Until recently, the direct impact of PD and of therapies on patients has been assessed by means of clinical scales of physical impairment. It has been suggested that these measures do not assess psychosocial factors which are important components of well-being and, in terms of patients' quality of life, are perhaps the most important outcome variables in treatment trials.[46] As this review has indicated, a range of instruments have now been shown to be of value in assessing a broader range of aspects of health-related quality of life in PD. Generic instruments have an important role in demonstrating the range of impacts of PD, because the results obtained can be compared to scores on the same instrument both for the general population and for other illness groups. Consequently, it is possible to 'norm' the data and interpret scores from specific patient groups with regard to the health of the population at large. Disease-specific questionnaires are more likely to be sensitive to the specific concerns of individuals with PD, and to be particularly appropriate for use in clinical trials. It is clear that the information obtained by such instruments directly complements the evidence obtained by conventional clinical scales, and it has been suggested that they should be used to evaluate treatment and long-term care regimes[47] where clinical measures provide only a limited view of the impact on the subjective experience of patients.

References

1 Sutcliffe R, Prior R, Mawby B and McQuillan W (1985) Parkinson's disease in the district of Northampton Health Authority, UK. A study of prevalence and disability. *Acta Neurol Scand.* **72**: 363–79.

2 Hoehn M and Yahr M (1967) Parkinsonism: onset, progression and mortality. *Neurology.* **17**: 427–42.

3 Hely M, Chey T, Wilson A *et al.* (1993) Reliability of the Columbia Scale for assessing signs of Parkinson's disease. *Mov Disord.* **8**: 466–72.

4 Fahn S, Elton RL and members of the UPDRS Development Committee (1987) Unified Parkinson's Disease Rating Scale. In: S Fahn, M Marsden, M Goldstein and DB Calne (eds) *Recent Developments in Parkinson's Disease. Volume 2.* MacMillan, New York.

5 Schwab RS and England AC (1969) Projection technique for evaluating surgery in Parkinson's disease. In: FJ Gillingham and MC Donaldson (eds) *Third Symposium on Parkinson's Disease.* Churchill Livingstone, Edinburgh.

6 Bryson H, Milne R and Chrisp P (1992) Selegiline: an appraisal of the basis of its pharmaco-economic and quality-of-life benefits in Parkinson's disease. *Pharmaco-economics.* **2**: 118–36.

7 Guyatt G and Cook D (1994) Health status, quality of life, and the individual. *JAMA.* **272**: 630–31.

8   Bowling A (1995) What things are important in people's lives? A survey of the public's judgements to inform scales of health-related quality of life. *Soc Sci Med.* **41**: 1447–62.

9   Bulpitt C, Shaw K, Clifton P, Stern G, Davies J and Reid J (1985) The symptoms of patients treated for Parkinson's disease. *Clin Neuropharmacol.* **8**: 175–83.

10 Quinn W and Oertel N (1997) Parkinson's disease drug therapy. *Ballières Clin Neurol.* **97**: 89–108.

11 Lees A, Blackburn N and Campbell V (1998) The night-time problems of Parkinson's disease. *Clin Neuropharmacol.* **11**: 512–19.

12 Mutch W, Strudwick A, Roy S and Downie A (1986) Parkinson's disease: disability, review and management. *BMJ.* **293**: 675–77.

13 Koller W and Vetere-Overfield B (1988) Falls and Parkinson's disease (abstract). *Ann Neurol.* **24**: 153–4.

14 Welburn P and Walker S (1988) Assessment of quality of life in Parkinson's disease. In: G Teeling Smith (ed.) *Measuring Health: A Practical Approach.* John Wiley & Sons, Chichester.

15 Longstreth W, Nelson L, Linde M and Munoz D (1992) Utility of the Sickness Impact Profile in Parkinson's disease. *J Geriatr Psychiatry Neurol.* **5**: 142–8.

16 Clarke C, Zobkiw R and Gullaksen E (1995) Quality of life and care in Parkinson's disease. *Br J Clin Pract.* **49**: 288–93.

17 Oxtoby M (1982) *Parkinson's Disease Patients and their Social Needs.* Parkinson's Disease Society, London.

18 Rubenstein L, Chrischilles E and Voelker M (1997) The impact of Parkinson's disease on health status, health expenditures and productivity. *Pharmaco-economics.* **12**: 486–98.

19 Shindler J, Brown R, Welburn P and Parkes J (1993) Measuring the quality of life of patients with Parkinson's disease. In: S Walker and R Rosser (eds) *Quality of Life Assessment: Key Issues in the 1990s.* Kluwer Academic Publishers, Dordrecht.

20   Gotham A, Brown R and Marsden C (1986) Depression in Parkinson's disease: a quantitative and qualitative analysis. *J Neurol Neurosurg Psychiatry.* **49**: 381–9.

21   Nijhof G (1995) Parkinson's disease as a problem of shame in public appearance. *Sociol Health Illness.* **17**: 193–205.

22   Bergner M, Bobbitt RA, Carter WB and Gilson B (1981) The Sickness Impact Profile: development and final revision of a health status measure. *Med Care.* **19**: 787–805.

23   Patrick D and Peach H (1989) *Disablement in the Community.* Oxford University Press, Oxford.

24   Hunt S, McEwen J and McKenna S (1986) *Measuring Health Status.* Croom Helm, London.

25   Ware J and Sherbourne C (1992) The MOS 36-Item Short-Form Health Survey. 1. Conceptual framework and item selection. *Med Care.* **30**: 473–83.

26   Pahwa R, Lyons K, McGuire D *et al.* (1977) Comparison of standard carbidopa-levodopa and sustained-release carbidopa-levodopa in Parkinson's disease: pharmacokinetic and quality-of-life measures. *Mov Disord.* **12**: 677–81.

27   Karlsen KH, Larsen PJ, Tandberg E and Maeland JG (1999) Influence of clinical and demographic variables on quality of life in patients with Parkinson's disease. *J Neurol Neurosurg Psychiatry.* **66**: 431–5.

28   Jenkinson C, Peto V, Fitzpatrick R, Greenhall R and Hyman N (1995) Self-reported functioning and well-being in patients with Parkinson's disease: a comparison of the Short-Form Health Survey (SF-36) and the Parkinson's Disease Questionnaire (PDQ-39). *Age Ageing.* **24**: 505–9.

29   Chrischilles EA, Rubenstein LM, Voelker MD, Wallace RB and Rodnitzky RL (1998) The health burdens of Parkinson's disease. *Mov Disord.* **13**: 406–13.

30   Mercer B (1996) A randomized study of the efficacy of the PROPATH programme for patients with Parkinson's disease. *Arch Neurol.* **53**: 881–4.

31 Hobson P and Meara J (1997) Self-reported functioning and well-being in patients with Parkinson's disease (letter to the editor). *Age Ageing.* **25**: 334–5.

32 Calne S, Schulzer M, Mak E *et al.* (1996) Validating a quality-of-life rating scale for idiopathic parkinsonism: Parkinson's Impact Scale (PIMS). *Parkinson Rel Disord.* **2**: 55–61.

33 De Boer AGEM, Wijker W, Speelman JD and de Haes J (1996) Quality of life in patients with Parkinson's disease: development of a questionnaire. *J Neurol Neurosurg Psychiatry.* **61**: 70–74.

34 Peto V, Jenkinson C, Fitzpatrick R and Greenhall R (1995) The development and validation of a short measure of functioning and well-being for individuals with Parkinson's disease. *Qual Life Res.* **4**: 241–8.

35 Jenkinson C, Fitzpatrick R and Peto V (1998) *The Parkinson's Disease Questionnaire. User Manual for the PDQ-39, PDQ-8 and PDQ Summary Index.* Health Services Research Unit, Oxford.

36 McDowell I and Jenkinson C (1996) Development standards for health measures. *J Health Serv Res Policy.* **1**: 238–46.

37 Damiano AM, Snyder C, Strausser B and Willian MK (1999) A review of health-related quality-of-life concepts and measures for Parkinson's disease. *Qual Life Res.* **8**: 235–43.

38 Hobson P, Holden A and Meara J (1999) Measuring the impact of Parkinson's disease with the Parkinson's Disease Quality of Life questionnaire. *Age Ageing.* **28**: 341–6.

39 Cronbach L (1951) Coefficient alpha and the internal structure of tests. *Psychometrica.* **16**: 297–334.

40 Carmines E and Zeller R (1979) *Reliability and Validity Assessment: Quantitative Applications in the Social Sciences.* Sage, Beverley Hills, CA.

41 Nunnally JC (1978) *Psychometric Theory* (2e). McGraw Hill, New York.

42 Fitzpatrick R, Peto V, Jenkinson C, Greenhall R and Hyman N (1997) Health-related quality of life in Parkinson's disease: a study of out-patient clinic attenders. *Mov Disord.* **6**: 916–22.

43 Martinez-Martin P, Frades Payo B and the Grupo Centro for Movement Disorders (1998) Quality of life in Parkinson's disease: validation study of the PDQ-39 Spanish version. *J Neurol.* **245** (**Supplement 1**): S34–8.

44 Cohen J (1977) *Statistical Power for the Behavioural Sciences.* Academic Press, New York.

45 Ware J, Kosinski M, Bayliss M, McHorney C, Rogers W and Raczek A (1995) Comparison of methods for the scoring and statistical analysis of SF-36 health profile and summary measures: summary of results from the Medical Outcomes Study. *Med Care.* **33**: AS264–79.

46 Martinez-Martin P, Frades Payo B, Fontan-Tirado C, Martinez Sarries FJ, Guerrero M and del Ser Quijano yT (1997) Valoracion de la calidad de vida en la enfermedad de Parkinson mediante el PDQ-39. Estudio piloto. *Neurologia.* **12**: 56–60.

47 Fukunaga H, Kasai T and Yoshidome H (1997) Clinical findings, status of care, comprehensive quality of life, daily life therapy and treatment at home in patients with Parkinson's disease. *Eur Neurol.* **38** (**Supplement 2**): 64–9.

4
Multiple sclerosis

Ray Fitzpatrick, Jeremy Hobart and Alan Thompson

Introduction

Multiple sclerosis (MS) is a chronic disorder of the central nervous system (the brain and spinal cord) in which there is damage to the protective myelin sheath that surrounds the nerve fibres (demyelination) and also loss of nerve fibres (axonal loss). This damage disrupts normal neurological function. Viral and immune causes have been postulated, and both genetic and environmental factors are also implicated.

There are two age peaks of onset of MS, namely in the twenties and in the forties, with females being more frequently affected than males. MS affects approximately 85 000 individuals in the UK and 1.1 million world-wide, with unexplained tendencies to be more common among Caucasians and those living in more northern and temperate latitudes.

Several different clinical courses have been identified for this disorder.

- Relapsing remitting MS (the commonest pattern) involves unpredictable relapses for varying periods of days or months, with partial or total remission.

- Secondary progressive MS involves a relapsing remitting pattern but with later progressive disability.

- Primary progressive MS is progressive without a history of clear-cut relapses or remission.

- Benign MS involves little or no disability after 15 years.

The symptoms are highly variable in severity, duration and nature. Motor symptoms include weakness of the hands, difficulties in walking, speech and swallowing, imbalance and poor co-ordination. Sensory symptoms include numbness, tingling and loss of sensation. Bladder symptoms include problems of frequency, urgency and incontinence, and bowel problems include urgency, incontinence and constipation. Cognitive problems include short-term memory loss, difficulty in concentrating and thinking, and disinhibition. Visual symptoms include blurred vision, decreased visual acuity, moving visual images, impaired perception of distance and speed. Because symptoms may be due to any of a number of conditions other than MS, the diagnosis may sometimes be protracted. It is a clinical diagnosis which is supported or confirmed by laboratory tests. Lumbar puncture is used to detect specific proteins that indicate an inflammatory disorder within the central nervous system. Evoked potentials measure nerve conduction times (which are reduced in demyelination) and the magnitude of the response to the stimulus (which is decreased when axons have been lost).

A number of therapeutic strategies may be employed for individuals with MS, although none of them are curative. For many years corticosteroids have been used to address exacerbations by reducing inflammation. However, over longer periods they are not effective. Moreover, they cannot be used for long periods because of potential side-effects and problems of immune suppression. More recently, a number of potentially disease-modifying drugs have been developed which are currently at various stages of testing. Interferon β-1b (injected subcutaneously) and β-1a (injected intramuscularly) have been shown to have some beneficial effects in reducing the relapse rate and the number of newly appearing lesions in the relapsing remitting form of MS. Their effects in terms of reducing the rate of worsening of disability are less clearly established. Interferon β-1a is thought to be less prone to exert the flu-like side-effects that can occur with interferon β-1b. More recently, Copaxone (injected subcutaneously) has appeared which has a different mode of action to interferon β and is also able to decrease the frequency of relapses in patients with relapsing remitting disease, with few severe side-effects. Other medications may be used for symptomatic relief of specific problems such as pain or bladder control.

Interventions from a range of health professionals are important to manage the consequences of MS at different stages of the disorder. Physiotherapists devise appropriate exercise programmes, while occupational therapists provide specific aids and equipment to reduce the difficulties of travel or functioning in the home that are caused by disability. Speech therapy is helpful for addressing speech and swallowing problems. Other interventions include advice about diet, a variety of treatment strategies for incontinence, and input from social workers about benefits and other social services. A multidisciplinary approach is therefore required for the rehabilitation of patients with the disorder.

Clinical assessment

Until recently, the outcomes of MS were measured entirely by clinical judgement. In almost all research contexts this has been carried out by means of Kurtzke's Expanded Disability Status Scale (EDSS).[1] The EDSS is a 20-point rating scale (from 0–10 with 0.5-point increments) which is based on ratings of disability for eight functional systems that are assessed during neurological examination (pyramidal, cerebellar, brainstem, sensory, bladder and bowel, visual, mental and other). A single score is obtained, with 0 signifying no disability and 10 indicating death.

The EDSS tends to generate data that are non-linear and with a bimodal distribution of scores at the top and bottom of the scale. Studies of inter-rater reliability have found poor levels of agreement, especially at the lower levels of the distribution.[2] There is serious concern about the lack of sensitivity of the scale to change, especially at the more severe end of the spectrum of disability, in which state many patients may expect to spend a prolonged period.[3] Above all, as will be seen in the evidence examined below, the EDSS does not address issues of concern to patients with MS, whether these are symptoms such as fatigue, or the broader psychosocial consequences of the disease.

As well as the long-established and widely used EDSS, scales developed in other contexts have been applied for use in MS. For example, the Functional Independence Measure (FIM) is an 18-item interviewer-based instrument originally designed to assess the level of assistance needed by patients receiving rehabilitation for problems such as stroke and head injury.[4] In a clinical series of patients with MS, the measurement properties of the EDSS were examined in relation to those of other clinical scales that are less commonly used in the assessment of outcomes of MS, such as the FIM.[5] The authors concluded that, when evidence of reliability, validity and responsiveness was considered together, no single measure dominated. Other evidence suggests substantially poorer responsiveness of the EDSS compared to other measures of MS.[6] The limitations of the available clinical scales have resulted in the recent development of the Multiple Sclerosis Functional Composite (MSFC), but this measure has not yet been extensively tested.[7] Although much criticised, the absence of superior clinical scales results in the EDSS tending to be recommended for neurological outcome assessment.[8]

One of the earliest studies to indicate the substantial capacity of patients themselves to provide accurate and meaningful information about disability arising from MS was conducted in France by investigators who drew up a 25-item questionnaire intended to provide patients' assessments of each of the eight dimensions distinguished in the EDSS scale.[9] The questionnaire used simple everyday language, and for each item patients were offered four response categories ranging from 'none' to 'severe'. For all dimensions except symptoms relating to brainstem function (e.g. speaking or swallowing) or mental function (e.g. memory or calculation), the levels of agreement between patients' responses to the questionnaire and neurologists' judgements on the EDSS were substantial ($r > 0.50$) and significant. The levels of agreement did not vary according to demographic or disease characteristics. The authors concluded that, although accuracy was not sufficient for such an approach to be relied on in decision-making for individual patients, by contrast, self-report by questionnaire was a promising method of measuring disability in MS for group and community level applications. The rest of this chapter describes the ways in which the approach of relying on patients' judgements rather than health professionals' assessments of health status in MS have developed from this early study.

Generic measures

Generic measures of health status are intended to be applicable to a wide range of health problems. One particular advantage is that they permit direct comparison of the benefits (in terms of health) of treatments across a wide spectrum of diseases. This is clearly an advantage where decisions have to be made about, for example, resource allocation in healthcare, taking into account the health gain obtained from interventions for widely differing health problems.

One of the first generic health status measures to be developed and widely applied was the Sickness Impact Profile (SIP).[10] The measure was designed to assess changes in a person's behaviour as a consequence of ill health. By focusing on the behavioural consequences of sickness, it was considered more readily verifiable than approaches that focus on feelings or perceptions. It consists of 136 statements with 'yes' or 'no' response categories and positively affirmed items weighted according to severity. Items are combined to provide scores in 12 categories, namely ambulation, mobility, body care and movement, social interaction, alertness, emotions, communication, sleep and rest, eating, work, home management, and recreation and pastimes. It is also possible to derive two summary scores (a physical summary score and a psychosocial summary score) as well as an overall global index. The instrument has been validated for a wide range of health problems.

The validity of the SIP for MS was examined in a series of 50 patients with clinically definite MS who completed the SIP as well as being assessed by the Expanded Disability Status Scale (EDSS) on two occasions separated by a period of 6 months.[11] On both occasions, correlations were significant between the SIP physical scale and the EDSS ($r = 0.77$ on both occasions). Reproducibility was examined by the change in scores on the SIP physical scale in patients assessed as remaining unchanged over time on the EDSS, and the mean level of change observed was less than 1 point. Sensitivity to change was examined by calculating the change in scores for those individuals who were clinically judged to have changed on EDSS, and it was found to be 8 points. The authors considered this to be promising evidence of sensitivity to change, in contrast to the EDSS. The correlations of EDSS with the psychosocial scale were 0.18 and 0.19 in the two assessments, and were regarded as evidence that this dimension is independent of physical disability. It is of interest that, although it is generally considered appropriate for self-completion, in this study the instrument was administered by interview (lasting 20 minutes on average). The authors suggest that this mode of administration may be necessary in cases where respondents experience problems in reading or hand function due to MS. The length of the SIP can be an important problem limiting its more widespread use.

Lankhorst *et al.* developed the self-administered Disability and Impact Profile (DIP) on the basis of the World Health Organisation's International Classification of Impairments, Disabilities and Handicaps.[12] It contains three symptom-focused questions and 36 disability-related questions in the domains of mobility, self-care, social activities, communication and psychological status. Respondents rate each item on a 10-point scale of extent of disability, and then again on extent of importance. The second item is used to weight the score provided by the first item, and it expresses the subjective impact on quality of life. The DIP was not originally designed to produce a single summed score or dimension scores. In a comparison of patients with MS, rheumatoid arthritis and spinal cord injury, significant differences between the three groups were observed for 22 out of 39 items, with patients with MS scoring particularly poorly in areas such as reading, memory and concentration. Subsequent analyses have shown that weighted scoring (i.e. using patients' ratings of importance) did not significantly alter patients' scores. The authors considered that, despite this finding, 'impact' should not therefore be dropped from the instrument.[13] A two-factor solution was also observed indicating two underlying scales – physical and psychological. With regard to construct validity, the physical scale, but not the psychological scale, was observed to correlate substantially (0.65) with the EDSS, whilst the psychological scale correlated significantly with a battery of other familiar and validated psychological measures. Although it has been used to compare different chronic illnesses, it appears to be intended to be of particular relevance to MS.

Another generic instrument that focuses specifically on disability is the Functional Status Questionnaire.[14] Like other instruments, it is intended to be self-completed and it consists of 34 items that are either independent or contribute to one of six scales, namely basic activities of daily living (ADL), intermediate ADL, mental health, work performance, social activity and quality of interaction. It has been tested in a number of areas of physical medicine and rehabilitation.

Murphy *et al.* examined its validity for patients with MS in France, Germany and the UK.[15] For the purposes of the study, basic and IADL scales were combined to form a physical function scale, and a social role function was produced by combining work, social activity and quality of interaction. Scores for all domains were found to be poorer for patients who were seen by a neurologist than for a control group of other patients consulting a doctor. Correlations were found to be high between EDSS and physical function, moderate for social function and low for mental health. The study also reports encouraging evidence of the internal consistency of scales, with a higher Cronbach's alpha for physical function than for social function.

It is not surprising that the most extensively studied generic measure for use in MS is the SF-36, as this instrument has been most widely tested and applied across most fields of healthcare.[16] It is a self-completed 36-item questionnaire with eight domains, namely physical functioning, role limitations due to physical problems, role limitations due to emotional problems, pain, social functioning, emotional well-being, energy and general health perceptions. Brunet *et al.* examined the level of agreement between SF-36 scales and EDSS scores completed by a neurologist for patients with MS attending a clinic in Canada.[17] Only one scale, namely physical functioning, correlated significantly with EDSS. A very similar result was reported by Rothwell *et al.*, who also found that only SF-36 physical functioning correlated significantly with EDSS in a series of MS patients attending neurology services.[18] They also compared scores with those expected from population normative data and found lower scores for all scales, and particularly poor values for patients with MS for physical functioning, physical role limitations, vitality, general health and mental health.

A larger Canadian study examined patients with MS attending one of 14 neurological clinics.[19] On all domains, SF-36 scores deteriorated with greater disease severity on the EDSS, but this trend was only significant for physical functioning, physical role limitations and social function. As with other studies, scores for all domains were poorer than those for a normative population, but they were markedly so for physical functioning, physical role limitations and social function. The study showed that even at the mildest level of EDSS disease severity, patients with MS had poorer scores for all dimensions of the SF-36 than the normative population, with physical role and vitality domains being most adversely affected (63% and 31% lower, respectively, than for a normal population of similar age). In their discussion, the authors raise an important issue. Noting that by comparison with physical function most other dimensions of health status do not decline so markedly with disease progression, they argue that it is difficult to determine whether such effects are due to patient adaptation or insensitivity of the SF-36.

A study of patients with MS in Norway also found poorer scores for all dimensions of the SF-36 compared to population norms, the differences being especially marked for physical functioning, physical role limitations, vitality and social functioning.[20] These dimensions also correlated most strongly with EDSS scores, but the correlations were particularly high (0.86) for physical functioning. There is evidence that the SF-36 is susceptible to floor effects when assessing physical function. For example, a study in the UK of patients with MS undergoing rehabilitation found that a substantial proportion of patients with the lowest possible score on the SF-36 physical function and physical role limitations scales reported a wide range of scores on other measures of disability.[21]

A distinctive approach that may be considered under the heading of generic measures is the so-called 'preference' or 'utility'-based approach to measuring patients' perceptions of their health problems. These terms are used to describe a particular approach which uniquely attempts to elicit the overall preferences ('utility' is a more technical term derived from economic theory) of a patient with regard to his or her health state and the balance of positive and negative aspects of treatment for that state. Other generic measures reviewed to date categorise patients' experiences according to distinct and separately measured dimensions of health status (e.g. physical, emotional and social aspects). Preference measures elicit the overall global value that respondents attach to a state, having made trade-offs between the various positive and negative aspects of health and treatment.

Schwartz et al. explored the preference approach in patients with MS by a method that focuses on Quality-Adjusted Time Without Symptoms and Toxicities (Q-Twist).[22,23] Essentially in the context of treatments for MS this approach requires that patients make judgements about their preferences with regard to possible therapeutic gains concerning disability and disease progression, traded off against the disadvantages of treatment side-effects. This produces an overall preference which is then used as a weighting or adjustment of time spent in a given state. To date, reports of this approach have not given clear descriptions of how preferences were elicited, and these reports have illustrated how the technique might be used, rather than producing clear results. In contrast to methods based on self-completed questionnaires, this approach requires trained interviewers and more time commitment by both investigators and respondents to participate in data collection.

Finally, among the generic approaches, mention should be made of the London Handicap Scale.[24] As its name suggests, it purports to assess the broader social, economic and other consequences of illness, in contrast to the emphasis of most measures reviewed in this chapter, which focus on impairment and disability. The core questionnaire asks respondents to choose which of six descriptions best applies to them for each of six areas of disadvantage arising from their health state. They are then required to complete visual analogue scales designed to elicit their personal preferences for such states. This measure has been applied to patients with MS receiving rehabilitation.[25] Whereas no differences were observed when using the EDSS scale, the London Handicap Scale showed significant benefits of rehabilitation.

Disease-specific measures

A major potential limitation in so-called generic measures is that they may fail to address issues of particular importance to specific diseases. Since, in research contexts such as clinical trials, investigators are seeking evidence of relatively small therapeutic benefits, it is important to test measures that have been specifically targeted at the disease under investigation. Therefore some considerable effort has recently been made by a number of research groups to produce measures that are more specifically relevant to the problems arising from MS.

Vickrey et al. adopted a strategy common to several of the measures that have emerged in this particular area, namely to adopt a well-established generic health status measure, in this case the SF-36, and to add on items of specific relevance to MS. This was done in two ways.[26] First, additional items were added to certain existing scales of the SF-36; individual items were added to the social function, pain and energy scales to reflect specific problems of MS (e.g. limitations in social function due to bladder or bowel function). Secondly, four new scales, namely health distress, overall quality of life, sexual function, and cognitive function, were added to the core SF-36. Items were identified both from literature review and from the expert opinion of health professionals. Internal reliability and reproducibility for the new instrument (referred to as QOL-54) were established to be satisfactory. Validity was examined by means of correlations with other self-reported items such as symptom severity, number of days unable to work and depressive symptoms. No evidence of responsiveness was reported. A substantial proportion of patients omit items on sexual function, suggesting that this scale may be unacceptable.

The approach of adding MS-specific items to an established measure was further explored by Vickrey *et al.* by means of a study in which patients with MS completed the SF-36 as well as three 'bolted-on' components intended to be targeted at MS.[27] The first component consisted of three of the scales identified in the study cited previously, namely health distress, sexual function and cognitive function. The second component was a hitherto relatively unexplored quality-of-life questionnaire for MS consisting of five scales – physical problems, mobility, fatigue, control and emotional upset. The third component added on to the core SF-36 consisted of two scales – an MS ADL scale and an MS Help From Others scale. The various additional components showed satisfactory internal consistency and reproducibility. Criterion variables were selected to examine construct validity, namely patients' self-reports of symptom severity, disability reflected in walking, depressive symptoms and overall self-rated quality of life. Regression analyses on these four criterion variables showed that the various MS-specific additional scales had statistically significant effects over and above the effects of core SF-36 scale scores. It was concluded that disease-targeted scales provide unique information that is not detected by the generic SF-36 measure. However, no single version of the additional MS-specific scales was clearly and consistently related to the criteria. Therefore it is not easy to infer from the study what final combination of SF-36 with additional MS-specific components is preferable.

Cella *et al.* also decided that, in order to produce a disease-specific measure, they should start from an existing validated measure.[28] They adopted the 28-item Functional Assessment of Cancer Therapy, General Version (FACT-G).[29] Patients with MS rated all items of this instrument as relevant to their condition. A total of 135 new items were added on to this core instrument in response to interviews with MS patients and health professionals. An expert panel then reduced the new items down to 60 questions on the basis of relevance or redundancy, thereby producing an instrument containing 88 items. Data from patients with MS were collected by means of this new instrument and then subjected to Rasch analysis and principal-components analysis. These analyses produced a 44-item instrument with six subscales, namely mobility, symptoms, emotional well-being, general contentment, thinking/fatigue and family/social well-being. A total of 15 original items were added back to the instrument as unscored independent items.

The new instrument (termed the Functional Assessment of Multiple Sclerosis or FAMS) was tested for internal consistency, reproducibility and construct validity with the EDSS and other health status instruments. The mobility scale was strongly correlated with the EDSS, but the other scales were not. The authors considered that correlations with other health status instruments provided evidence in support of the construct validity of the other scales of the FAMS.

The authors argue that the weak association of scales other than mobility with the EDSS is evidence of the additional information provided by the new instrument. Scales such as fatigue address an important aspect of MS that is not covered by many other instruments. The authors also argue that it is advantageous that the instrument has embedded within it an instrument for assessing patients' quality of life in cancer, because it permits direct comparison between the two diseases.

Fischer et al. developed an instrument known as the Multiple Sclerosis Quality of Life Inventory (MSQLI) along similar principles to those used to develop the QOL-54 and FAMS. An established and validated measure, in this case the SF-36, was adopted as the core of the instrument.[30] However, it was decided that instead of developing new additional items to be relevant to individuals with MS, the extra items added should also comprise scales that had already been validated. It was argued that the advantage would be that comparisons with other diseases could be made not only by means of the core instrument, but also with the additional components. Three expert panels composed of neurologists, other health professionals, and patients and caregivers examined candidate validated scales and eventually selected scales in nine areas, namely fatigue, pain, sexual function, bladder function, bowel function, visual function, cognitive function, emotional status and social relationships, to be added to the SF-36. The resulting instrument consisted of 137 items, although the authors report (from data yet to be published) that an abbreviated 80-item version was derived. The instrument was examined for psychometric properties and correlation with other measures such as the EDSS, and it was reported that the observed relationships were satisfactory. As with other studies of the components of the MSQLI, the physical function scale correlated most strongly with the EDSS.

Full analyses of the MSQLI have yet to be reported. However, the authors claim that, compared to other instruments, it is more comprehensive and relevant to patients with MS, as it has assessments of key issues for patients with MS (e.g. visual, bladder and bowel problems). However, they also acknowledge that it is over twice as long as instruments such as the QOL-54, and requires about 45 minutes to complete.

In a very similar vein, Pfennings et al. also set out to develop a quality-of-life questionnaire for use in MS, based on established validated instruments.[31] They administered to patients with MS an instrument consisting of the SF-36, the COOP Charts[32] and the Disability and Impact Profile (DIP, discussed above) in a longitudinal study conducted over 6 months. Factor analyses identified two underlying dimensions – physical and psychological. The three highest-loading scales for each of the two factors were then identified and confirmed by further factor analyses. An instrument emerged with 26 items consisting of physical functioning, with three contributing scales (mobility, self-care and physical functioning) and 14 items consisting of psychological functioning, with three contributing scales (mental health, psychological status and vitality). The six constituent scales appear to correspond largely in content with the original scales of the SF-36 and DIP. As with many other analyses of instruments in this field, correlations with the EDSS were greater with physical functioning than with psychological functioning.

The final instrument requires about 10 minutes to complete, and this relative brevity is considered by its authors to be an advantage. They also argue that the inclusion of content from the DIP (e.g. ability to stand, reach, use the hands and eat) should mean that the instrument is less prone to floor effects in MS that might prevail with SF-36 physical functioning. They note that the new instrument does not contain a social dimension. This may be due to the fact that there is no unique variance apart from physical and psychological functioning.

Finally, Schwartz *et al.* set out to develop patient-reported neurological impairment and disability scales.[33] In other words, it was not their intention to capture broader aspects of health-related quality of life. They proceeded by drawing up two sets of items, one of symptoms (the Symptom Inventory, with alternative long 99-item and short 29-item versions) and one of disability (Performance Scales, 8 items) on the basis of clinical experience. The Symptom Inventory addresses issues that are described in terms such as visual, left hemisphere, right hemisphere, spinal cord problems, whereas the Performance Scales address issues such as mobility, hand function, fatigue, cognitive and bladder/bowel problems. The resulting instruments were then pretested with focus groups of patients with MS and subsequently examined for validity in a cross-sectional study of patients with MS and a healthy control group. Internal consistency and reproducibility were tested and found to be satisfactory. Corrrelations with clinical assessment of the EDSS and of ambulation and cane use were considered to provide evidence in support of construct validity. Although the two measures correlated substantially, they explained only small amounts of the additional variance of other clinical measures when used together compared to either used alone, and were therefore considered to make only small unique contributions of information about patients, so it was assumed that they did not need to be used simultaneously in trials.

Discussion

It is difficult not to relate the relative explosion of patient-assessed outcome measures in MS from the latter half of the 1990s to the emergence in 1993 of interferon β-1b. Potentially important advances in the drug treatment of MS have made the need for appropriate and valid measures of outcomes that are of concern to patients with MS a priority.

Much of what has emerged since the mid-1990s is highly encouraging. For example, in the many generic and disease-specific approaches that have been developed, there is substantial convergence with regard to the health concerns to be assessed in individuals with MS. In the field of physical disability there is considerable agreement, not only about which topics of importance need to be assessed (e.g. walking, rising, self-care and related domains of physical function), but also about the considerable accuracy with which patients can report such domains. Instruments converge in their repeated emphasis in other areas as well – for example, the importance of physical symptoms, bowel and bladder control, problems of speech, communication and vision, and a spectrum of cognitive and psychological responses to MS. There is less convergence in broader areas such as social function, although the field is no different in this respect from health status measurement in other fields.[34]

The evolution of approaches to the measurement of patients' perspectives with regard to MS is unusual in one particular aspect. Many of the instruments that have emerged have built upon existing validated instruments. It is understandable that investigators should not seek to 'reinvent the wheel' in developing measures for MS. Nevertheless, it is unusual for disease-specific measures to be developed in this way, given the growing recognition of the importance of identifying the content of disease-specific health status questionnaires by maximal input at all stages of development of individuals who have the relevant condition.[35] Partly because of the need for instruments with very wide-ranging applicability, instruments such as the

SF-36 were developed with a somewhat different methodology, relying more on expert opinion to identify items of health status of broad applicability. There is therefore still scope for the development and testing of instruments that are more firmly and explicitly based on evidence of the experiences and assessments of individuals with MS.

In just a short time the field has adopted psychometric methods to an impressive degree in order to assess the applicability of both new and established instruments to MS. Substantial evidence of reliability, reproducibility and validity has been presented for most of the instruments described in this chapter. It is now clear that many aspects of the outcomes of interventions for MS can be evaluated with as much if not greater accuracy by asking the patient as by relying on conventional neurological measures.[36] However, it is far less common for instruments to have been assessed in terms of sensitivity to change (responsiveness). This is a central property of instruments that is required to detect sometimes subtle therapeutic effects. As responsiveness has also been acknowledged to be a problem with clinical scales in this area, it is essential that more attention is given to this aspect of patient-based measures. In particular, given the widespread use of the SF-36 either by itself or in an adapted form, the frequent suggestion that instruments such as the SF-36 have significant 'floor effects' with regard to physical function requires further examination.[19,21,31] An essential requirement of instruments in this area is to detect deterioration at the most servere end of the spectrum of disability.

Three types of development are now required in the field of assessment of measures of outcome for MS from the patient's perspective. First, evidence is required from direct 'head-to-head' comparisons of the available alternative measures. Currently, instruments are largely reported in isolation of each other. Such comparative evaluation needs to take into account not only measurement properties such as reliability, validity and responsiveness, but also the acceptability and feasibility of use of alternative instruments as reflected by response rate and levels of incomplete data. There may well be 'trade-offs' between, on the one hand, the richness and extensiveness of data regarding patients' experiences from longer measures, and on the other, approaches that by their brevity ensure minimal burden and high response rates.[37] Secondly, methodological work is required to determine the effects of particular problems such as cognitive difficulties in influencing the responses of individuals with MS to questionnaires. Thirdly and most importantly, more evidence of the performance of instruments in clinical trials and evaluative research is required. To date, few major trials – whether of recently developed drugs or of rehabilitation programmes – have reported patient-assessed outcome measures. Not only does this make the assessment of the value of instruments difficult, but it also means that the research and clinical community continue to lack evidence with which to interpret the meaning of scores produced by this new approach to measurement. This in turn makes it more difficult to incorporate evidence from patients' values and assessments more fully into decision-making.

References

1 Kurtzke J (1983) Rating neurologic impairment in multiple sclerosis: an Expanded Disability Status Scale (EDSS). *Neurology*. **33**: 1444–52.

2 Nosworthy J, Vandervoort M, Wong C and Ebers G (1990) Inter-rater variability with the Expanded Disability Status Scale (EDSS) and Functional Systems (FS) in a multiple sclerosis clinical trial. *Neurology*. **40**: 971–5.

3 European Study Group on Interferon β-1b in Secondary Progressive MS (1998) Placebo-controlled multicentre randomised trial of interferon β-1b in treatment of secondary progressive multiple sclerosis. *Lancet*. **352**: 1491–7.

4 Granger C and Hamilton B (1992) UPS report: the Uniform Data System for Medical Rehabilitation. Report of first admissions for 1990. *Am J Phys Med Rehabil.* **71**: 108–13.

5 Sharrack B, Hughes RA, Soudain S and Dunn G (1999) The psychometric properties of clinical rating scales used in multiple sclerosis. *Brain.* **122**: 141–59.

6 Hobart J, Freeman J and Thompson A (2000) Kurtzke scales revisited: the application of psychometric methods to clinical intuition. *Brain.* In press.

7 Cutter GR, Baier ML, Rudick RA *et al.* (1999) Development of a multiple sclerosis functional composite as a clinical trial outcome measure. *Brain.* **122**: 871–82.

8 Rudick R, Antel J, Confavreux C *et al.* (1997) Recommendations from the National Multiple Sclerosis Society Clinical Outcomes Assessment Task Force. *Ann Neurol.* **42**: 379–82.

9 Verdier-Taillefer M, Roullet E, Cesaro P and Alperovitch A (1994) Validation of self-reported neurological disability in multiple sclerosis. *Int J Epidemiol.* **23**: 148–54.

10 Bergner M, Bobbitt R, Carter W and Gibson B (1981) The Sickness Impact Profile: development and final revision of a health status measure. *Med Care.* **19**: 789–805.

11 Hutchinson J and Hutchinson M (1995) The Functional Limitations Profile may be a valid, reliable and sensitive measure of disability in multiple sclerosis. *J Neurol.* **242**: 650–7.

12 Lankhorst G, Jelles F, Smits R *et al.* (1996) Quality of life in multiple sclerosis: the Disability and Impact Profile (DIP). *J Neurol.* **243**: 469–74.

13 Cohen L, Pouwer F, Pfennings L, Lankhorst G, van der Ploeg H and Polman C (1999) Factor structure of the Disability and Impact Profile in patients with multiple sclerosis. *Qual Life Res.* **8**: 141–50.

14 Jette A, Davies A, Cleary P *et al.* (1986) The Functional Status Questionnaire; reliability and validity when used in primary care. *J Gen Intern Med.* **1**: 143–9.

15 Murphy N, Confavreux C, Haas J *et al.* (1998) Quality of life in multiple sclerosis in France, Germany and the United Kingdom. *J Neurol Neurosurg Psychiatry.* **65**: 460–66.

16 Ware J and Sherbourne C (1992) The MOS 36-item Short Form health survey (SF-36). 1. Conceptual framework and item selection. *Med Care.* **30**: 473–83.

17 Brunet D, Homan W, Singer M, Edgar C and MacKenzie T (1996) Measurement of health-related quality of life in multiple sclerosis patients. *Can J Neurol Sci.* **23**: 99–103.

18 Rothwell P, McDowell Z, Wong C and Dorman P (1997) Doctors and patients don't agree: cross-sectional study of patients' and doctors' perceptions and assessments of disability in multiple sclerosis. *BMJ.* **314**: 1580–3.

19 The Canadian Burden of Illness Study Group (1998) Burden of illness of multiple sclerosis. Part II. Quality of life. *Can J Neurol Sci.* **25**: 31–8.

20 Nortvedt M, Riise T, Kjell-Morten M and Nyland H (1999) Quality of life in multiple sclerosis: measuring the disease effects more broadly. *Neurology.* **53**: 1098–103.

21 Freeman J, Langdon D, Hobart J and Thompson A (1996) Health-related quality of life in people with multiple sclerosis undergoing inpatient rehabilitation. *J Neurol Rehabil.* **10**: 185–94.

22 Schwartz C, Cole B and Gelber R (1995) Measuring patient-centred outcomes in neurologic disease. *Arch Neurol.* **52**: 754–62.

23 Schwartz C, Coulthard-Morris I and Vollmer T (1997) The quality-of-life effects of interferon β-1b. *Arch Neurol.* **54**: 1475–80.

24 Harwood R, Rogers A, Dickinson E and Ebrahim S (1994) Measuring handicap. The London Handicap Scale: a new outcome measure for chronic disease. *Qual Health Care.* **3**: 11–16.

25 Freeman J, Langdon D, Hobart J and Thompson A (1997) The impact of inpatient rehabilitation on progressive mutliple sclerosis. *Arch Neurol.* **42**: 236–44.

26 Vickrey B, Hays R, Harooni R, Myers L and Ellison G (1995) A health-related quality-of-life measure for multiple sclerosis. *Qual Life Res.* **4**: 187–206.

27 Vickrey B, Hays R, Genovese B, Myers L and Ellison G (1997) Comparison of a generic to disease-targeted health-related quality-of-life measures for multiple sclerosis. *Clin Epidemiol.* **50**: 557–69.

28 Cella D, Dineen K, Arnason B *et al.* (1996) Validation of the Functional Assessment of Multiple Sclerosis quality of life instrument. *Neurology.* **47**: 129–39.

29 Cella D, Tulsky D, Gray G *et al.* (1993) The Functional Assessment of Cancer Therapy (FACT) Scale: development and validation of the general measure. *J Clin Oncol.* **11**: 570–79.

30 Fischer J, LaRocca N, Miller D, Ritvo P, Andrews H and Paty D (1999) Recent developments in the assessment of quality of life in multiple sclerosis (MS). *Mult Scler.* **5**: 251–9.

31 Pfennings L, Van der Ploeg H, Cohen L *et al.* (1999) A health-related quality-of-life questionnaire for multiple sclerosis patients. *Acta Neurol Scand.* **100**: 148–55.

32 Scholten J and van Weel C (1992) *Functional Status Assessment in Family Practice. The Dartmouth COOP Functional Health Assessment Charts/WONCA.* Meditekst, Lelystad.

33 Schwartz C, Vollmer T, Lee H and the North American Research Consortium on Multiple Sclerosis Outcomes Study Group (1999) Reliability and validity of two self-report measures of impairment and disability for MS. *Neurology.* **52**: 63–70.

34 Fitzpatrick R, Ziebland S, Jenkinson C, Mowat A and Mowat A (1991) The social dimension of health status measures in rheumatoid arthritis. *Int Disabil Stud.* **13**: 34–7.

35 Thompson A and Hobart J (1998) Multiple sclerosis: assessment of disability and disability scales. *J Neurol.* **245**: 189–96.

36 Rothwell P (1998) Quality of life in multiple sclerosis. *J Neurol Neurosurg Psychiatry.* **65**: 433.
37 Fitzpatrick R, Davey C, Buxton M and Jones D (1998) Evaluating patient-based outcome measures for use in clinical trials. *Health Technol Assess.* **2**: 1–74.

5
Stroke

Damian Jenkinson

Introduction and epidemiology of stroke

For the purposes of this review, the definition of stroke will be that used by the World Health Organisation – that is, 'a syndrome of rapidly developing clinical signs of focal (or global) disturbance of cerebral function, with symptoms lasting 24 hours or longer or leading to death, with no apparent cause other than of vascular origin'.[1] This is the definition that most epidemiological studies have used, and consequently it is likely that the total burden of stroke has been underestimated, as silent cerebral infarction has not been included.

Stroke is the most common cause of serious disability,[2] and the third most common cause of death.[3] Around 10–12% of deaths in the UK are due to stroke, and 88% of stroke deaths occur in those over 65 years of age.[4] Although there has been a decline in stroke mortality during the twentieth century, the reasons for this remain largely unexplained, indicating the current lack of knowledge of the risk factors for stroke.

The overall incidence of stroke is about 2.4 per 1000 members of the population per year in the UK.[5] One in four men and one in five women aged 45 years can expect to have a stroke if they live to 85 years.[6] The incidence of stroke is generally higher among populations in Eastern than in Western Europe.[7]

Stroke incidence rates rise exponentially with age, with a 100-fold increase from the fourth to the ninth decade of life. As the number of elderly people is increasing, it has been crudely estimated that over the next 30 years there will be a 30% increase in the incidence of stroke as a result of the ageing population.[7]

The proportion of people who have died one month after stroke depends on the age structure and health status of the population studied, and in the Oxford Community Stroke Project (OCSP) it has been reported to be 19% overall.[8] About half of the deaths within the first month are due to the direct neurological sequelae of the stroke, and after 30 days, non-stroke cardiovascular disease becomes increasingly important and is the most common cause of death after the first year.[9] The 1-year case fatality rate in the OCSP Study was 31%, and the 5-year survival rate was 55%.

One year after stroke, 35% of survivors are not functionally independent,[5] but these studies have not described the resultant disability adequately. One descriptive study estimated at three months that, of the survivors, 75% were able to walk out of doors, 20% were able to use public transport and only 12% were able to drive a car.[10]

Symptoms of stroke

The differentiation of stroke from a non-stroke diagnosis is accurate in more than 95% of cases if there is a clear history (from the patient or carer) of *focal* brain dysfunction of *sudden* onset, and if there is a residual *relevant* focal neurological deficit at the time of the clinical examination.[11,12] The physical functions that are affected by stroke reflect the area of the brain that has been damaged and the extent of the damage. About 30% of patients present with alteration to or loss of consciousness as their major clinical feature, and about 45% of non-comatose patients are confused in the initial stages.[13,14]

Paralysis (hemiplegia) or weakness (hemiparesis) of one side is the most obvious symptom and sign of stroke, occurring in 50–78% of cases. Weakness usually affects one side of the body, and crossed weakness suggests a brainstem or multifocal disturbance. Movement disorders with hemiballismus, unilateral asterixis, hemichorea and focal dystonia are uncommon recognised manifestations of deep-seated vascular lesions in the basal ganglia.

Unilateral sensory symptoms are less common (occurring in around 25% of non-comatose patients) and are usually associated with motor symptoms, but they may occur in isolation. The anatomical distribution of sensory symptoms is usually unilateral, affecting the face, arm and/or leg as is the case for motor symptoms.

It is difficult to be certain about the frequency of language disturbance, which is often misdiagnosed as confusion. The American National Survey of Stroke[13] suggested that 60% of all strokes had some language impairment, with around half of these describing slurred speech (dysarthria) and the other half experiencing difficulty in understanding or expressing spoken or written language (dysphasia). In a mute patient, it is important to ascertain whether it is a dysphasic or a dysarthric problem. This can be difficult in the acute stage and, of course, dysphasia and dysarthria may coexist.

Swallowing difficulties (dysphagia) are a common feature of acute stroke, with up to 45% of patients admitted to hospital showing some evidence of aspiration when asked to drink a small volume of water.[15] Estimates of the frequency of swallowing difficulty vary considerably because of differences in definitions, methods used for detecting dysphagia and the selection of patients. Furthermore, it is well recognised that aspiration may be 'silent'.[16]

Visual symptoms occur in around 7% of patients with acute stroke, and consist of visual loss confined to one eye, visual loss in both eyes, or double vision. It is important to determine whether visual disturbance involves one or both eyes. Isolated homonymous hemianopia (i.e. where the visual field to one side of the body is restricted in both eyes) is an uncommon symptom but a common sign in stroke patients, so it is essential to check the visual fields. Visual hallucinations may rarely occur after acute stroke.

The symptoms of isolated vertigo, ataxia, dysarthria, diplopia or dysphagia should not be regarded as definite symptoms of brainstem ischaemia. Patients who have suffered a genuine cerebrovascular event would usually have other symptoms and signs in association. Headache occurs in about 25% of patients with acute ischaemic stroke, in about 50% of patients with intra-cranial haemorrhage and in nearly all patients with subarachnoid haemorrhage.[17] About 2% of patients have an epileptic seizure at the onset of stroke; 50% of these are generalised and 50% are partial seizures.[18]

Treatment and rehabilitation

The goals of healthcare for stroke are as follows:

- to reduce the incidence of stroke by preventative methods
- to reduce case fatality once the stroke has occurred
- to reduce the level of disability due to stroke
- to help disabled patients to achieve their maximum functional potential
- to define the needs of those who remain permanently disabled
- to contribute to those needs
- to implement secondary prevention strategies to reduce the risk of a further vascular event.[19]

This section reviews those treatments for stroke for which there is now reasonable evidence of effectiveness, namely stroke units, aspirin, thrombolysis and some secondary prevention strategies.[20]

A recent meta-analysis of 19 well-designed studies[21] involving 3246 patients demonstrated that, compared to conventional care in a general medical ward, organised care in a stroke unit reduced the death rate by 17% ($P < 0.05$), reduced death and dependency by 31% ($P < 0.001$) and reduced death and institutionalisation by 25% ($P < 0.001$). These beneficial effects appeared to be independent of patients' age or sex or stroke severity. In the majority of these trials, stroke care was provided in a designated area or ward, as opposed to an ambulatory stroke care team. The practical implication of this is that acute in-patient care for patients with major stroke should be organised as a multidisciplinary stroke service based in designated units. The 1996 Declaration of Helsingborg called for organisation of stroke care by a multidisciplinary service,[22] and stated that an identified clinician with a special interest in stroke should have overall responsibility for the service. Multidisciplinary care should include involvement by medical, nursing, physiotherapy, occupational therapy, speech and language therapy, dietetics, social work and psychology staff, although there is a lack of evidence regarding the impact of these individual disciplines on outcomes after stroke.

Aspirin at a dose of 160–300 mg daily reduces the rate of death and dependency after acute ischaemic stroke from 47% to 45.8%.[23] Aspirin could theoretically be given to 95% of all stroke patients and protect about 1.8% from death or dependency, which is equivalent to a cost of about £177 to prevent one event.[20]

Intravenous thrombolysis within 6 hours of onset of ischaemic stroke may reduce the rate of death and dependency from 62.7% to 56.4%.[24] However, at present thrombolysis is likely to be accessible to or appropriate for only up to 10% of all cases of stroke, the remainder being excluded by delay between stroke onset and hospital admission, contraindications to thrombolysis, and difficulty in obtaining a computerised tomographic

(CT) scan to rule out intracranial haemorrhage. It has been estimated that the total cost of preventing one person from dying or becoming dependent using intravenous thrombolysis is £6816.[20]

The secondary prevention strategies for which there is reasonable evidence of effectiveness are control of vascular risk factors, antiplatelet drugs, anticoagulants and carotid endarterectomy. Lowering of the blood pressure of hypertensive stroke patients by 5–6 mmHg diastolic pressure and 10–12 mmHg systolic pressure for two to three years should reduce their annual risk of stroke from 7% to 4.8%.[25] Observational studies suggest that smoking increases the risk of transient ischaemic attack (TIA) and stroke at least 1.5-fold,[26] and although there are no randomised controlled trials for TIA and stroke patients, probably about 3.5% of all strokes could be avoided by the cessation of smoking.

As secondary prevention, aspirin given to TIA and ischaemic stroke patients in doses above 75 mg daily reduces the relative risk of stroke and other important vascular events by about 13%.[27] In patients with more widespread symptomatic vascular disease (e.g. ischaemic heart disease and peripheral vascular disease), aspirin reduces the relative risk of important vascular events by about 22%.[27] A total of 53 TIA and stroke patients need to be treated with aspirin at a cost of £2258 for one year in order to prevent one stroke.

Long-term oral anticoagulation for TIA and ischaemic stroke patients in atrial fibrillation reduces the annual risk of stroke from 12% to 4%.[28] However, only about 25% of suitable patients are actually treated. Anticoagulation of 12 TIA or ischaemic stroke patients will cost at least £2556 in order to prevent one stroke in a year.

Finally, carotid endarterectomy in highly selected patients reduces the 3-year risk of stroke from 26.5% to 14.9%.[29] The cost of carotid endarterectomy in 26 patients is about £387 660 in order to avoid one stroke each year for the following three years.

From the above, it can be seen that a treatment with a substantial effect on stroke outcome (e.g. thrombolysis) can have no more overall effect in the population than a much weaker treatment (e.g. aspirin) unless it can be given to more than a small minority of patients. At present, organised rehabilitation in stroke units is the only intervention that is appropriate for all patients. Greater potential for reducing the burden of stroke in the population may be offered by effective prevention.

Clinical measurement in stroke

There are many well-developed measures of stroke severity which can be divided into two broad groups, namely those which address a specific aspect of physical impairment (e.g. motor deficit in a limb) and those measures which mix a variety of impairments to provide a global measure of disease severity. Stroke has been studied sufficiently well for the individual determinants of prognosis to be well established, and in this regard the more specific measures are better validated. However, as research into short-term treatments in acute stroke has expanded, a number of stroke scales have been developed primarily for detecting therapeutic effect and matching of treatment groups in stroke trials. Both the measures of individual impairment and the global mixed indices will be considered briefly here.

A clinical system for making an accurate anatomical and pathophysiological diagnosis has been devised.[30] The Bamford Classification of Stroke identifies four subtypes of stroke on the basis of clinical features (total anterior circulation syndrome, partial anterior circulation syndrome, posterior circulation syndrome and lacunar syndrome). These syndromes predict the volume of cerebral infarction and, not surprisingly, they also predict outcome in terms of mortality and dependency. In addition, they provide an indication of the most likely underlying vascular pathology.

Clinical systems for distinguishing between haemorrhage and infarction have been devised.[31,32] However, the clinical differentiation of ischaemic stroke from haemorrhage will be incorrect in up to 10% of patients, and therefore brain imaging with CT or magnetic resonance imaging (MRI) is required in order to make this distinction reliably.

There is good evidence that motor loss is of great prognostic importance. The Motricity Index is a short, simple measure of motor loss developed primarily for use after stroke. Its validity and reliability have been demonstrated, and it is sensitive to change during recovery.[33] Other impairments can be measured using the Glasgow Coma Scale (level of consciousness), the Frenchay Aphasia Screening Test (communication), the Star Cancellation Test (neglect) and the Hodkinson Mental Test (confusion).

When measuring physical disability after stroke, there are many activities of daily living (ADL) scales available, but the best validated and most widely used is the Barthel Index.[34] The latter comprises the 10 most common areas included within ADL scales, and specifically covers continence of bowels and bladder, which some indices omit. The Barthel Index is extremely simple to use, taking only two or three minutes to complete. However, it does have definite floor and (more importantly) ceiling effects, and it is insensitive to small changes.

The Rankin Scale[35] is used as a measure of handicap, although it is strongly based on mobility and it mixes impairments with disabilities. This instrument is useful as an extremely simple outcome measure in large multicentre trials, but its sensitivity is low.[36]

A number of major stroke scales are used to detect therapeutic effect in stroke trials, but only the Middle Cerebral Artery Neurological Scale (MCANS),[37] the National Institute of Health Stroke Scale (NIHSS),[38] the Hemispheric Stroke Scale (HSS)[39] and the European Stroke Scale (ESS)[40] indicate the type of stroke for which the scale was intended. The MCANS omits certain important prognostic factors, such as visual field defects.

The inter-rater reliability of many stroke scales has not been adequately investigated, and only in the case of the Scandinavian Stroke Scale (SSS)[41] and the ESS are acceptable data available demonstrating good inter-rater reliability in terms of kappa statistics. In a direct comparison, the ESS was found to be more sensitive than the MCANS and the SSS, in that it distinguishes a greater number of steps in the recovery of neurological function after stroke.[40]

Health status measurement in stroke

Trials of treatment for acute stroke have primarily used measures of impairment and disability, as discussed in the preceding section, to assess the effect of treatment on outcome. However, these measures do not take into account psychological and social difficulties – outcomes which may be even more relevant to patients, and indeed which might not parallel physical outcomes either qualitatively or quantitatively.

In recognition of these deficiencies, clinical trials are increasingly including patient-centred outcomes such as health-related quality of life (HRQOL). HRQOL is broadly conceptualised as the physical, psychological and social aspects of life that can be affected by changes in health states.[42] HRQOL can be assessed with either generic or disease-specific measures. Generic measures are designed to compare HRQOL across populations of different diseases, whereas disease-specific measures are designed to assess HRQOL using questions and scales which are specific to a disease or condition.

Assessment of HRQOL in stroke is difficult, as patients have heterogeneous symptoms and deficits but at the same time suffer from psychological and social sequelae, and consequently experience with generic HRQOL measures after stroke is much greater than that with stroke-specific measures. These two groups of measures will be discussed in the following two sections.

Application of generic patient-based measures

Information regarding quality of life in stroke survivors is needed for both clinical practice and research, for the purpose of establishing baseline data, for setting goals, and for monitoring the success of interventions. There are two broad types of HRQOL measures — first, health status profiles that provide a series of scores, one for each dimension of a patient's health status, and secondly, single index measures which summarise the responses to all questions on every dimension of health state into a single index figure of health status. Multidimensional health status profiles which have been assessed in stroke patients include the Nottingham Health Profile (NHP),[43] the Sickness Impact Profile (SIP)[44] the Short Form 36 General Health Survey Questionnaire (SF-36)[45] and the Short Form 12 General Health Survey Questionnaire (SF-12).[46]

Examples of single index measures that are assessed in stroke patients include the EuroQol,[47] the Health Utilities Index (HUI)[48] and the Quality of Well-Being Scale.[49] The best validated measures of the profile type and of the single index type will be discussed below.

The SF-36 instrument[50] is designed to measure the impact of disease or disability of patients in eight dimensions (physical functioning, physical role limitations, bodily pain, general health, vitality, social functioning, emotional role limitations and mental health) on a scale of 0–100, using a 36-item questionnaire. Two core dimensions of health, namely physical and mental health, can be derived from these eight scales, and there is also a single item to assess change in health from one year previously. The questionnaire has already been subjected to substantial validation for use in the UK, and population norms exist for this measure.[51,52] The Australian version of the SF-36 was tested in 90 consecutive 1-year stroke survivors, with the instrument administered by personal interview.[45] Validity was assessed by comparing patients' scores on the SF-36 with those obtained for the Barthel Index, the General Health Questionnaire (GHQ) and the Adelaide Activities Profile (an instrument developed from the Frenchay Activities Index). The SF-36 appeared to be relatively quick and easy to use, and had satisfactory internal consistency (Cronbach's alpha <0.7). The SF-36 was correlated with physical disability defined by the Barthel Index and with emotional ill health defined by the GHQ, suggesting its validity for use in measuring physical and mental health. The SF-36 seemed to avoid the 'ceiling' effect of most disability scales, but it did not appear to characterise social functioning well, as measured by the Adelaide Activities Profile. No attempt was made by these authors to evaluate the sensitivity of the SF-36 to change in stroke patients.

An abbreviated version of the SF-36, the SF-12, has recently been developed.[53] The SF-12 generates the physical and mental component summary scores of the SF-36 with considerable accuracy, whilst imposing less burden on respondents. Evidence of the replicability of SF-36 scores by the SF-12 have been demonstrated in various patient subgroups, and was recently assessed using a telephone interview at 6 months after discharge in 162 stroke patients.[46] In this study, the SF-12 mental component summary scores and the SF-12 physical component summary scores were strongly correlated with the corresponding SF-36 summary scores for surveys completed both by proxy and by self-report (intra-class correlation coefficients were in the range 0.954–0.973). However, the mental health summary scores obtained by proxy assessment were strongly influenced by patient age, and thereby limited the replicability of the SF-36 by the SF-12 for older patients. The authors concluded that the SF-12 is an appropriate substitute for the SF-36 in stroke survivors who are capable of self-report, and possibly in proxy respondents when the eight subscale scores of the SF-36 are not sought.

The NHP is often regarded as a measure of general perceived health status, but the profile has been used in several stroke trials as a measurement of HRQOL[43,54] the NHP being a questionnaire consisting of two sections. The first section, which contains 38 items, is intended to measure perceptions of ill health. The items are distributed between the areas of pain (8 items), physical mobility (8 items), emotional reactions (9 items), sleep disturbance (5 items), social isolation (5 items) and energy (3 items). The second section asks respondents to indicate whether or not their state of health affects activity in seven areas of everyday life, namely job or work, looking after the house, social life, home life, sex life, interests and hobbies and holidays. The NHP has been utilised extensively in the general population and in various disease states, but there has been little research validating its usage in patients after stroke. NHP emotion scores correlated with objective measures of disability, length of hospital stay and scores from more complicated mood questionnaires in patients 6 months after stroke,[43] and the NHP appeared to be a valid indication of depressed mood, as combining its components into a total score gave the greatest accuracy in detecting depression. Indredavik *et al.* assessed 220 patients five years after stroke, of whom 110 patients had been allocated to a stroke unit and 110 patients to general medical wards in a randomised fashion.[54] Assessment with the NHP showed better results in the stroke unit group for the dimensions of energy, physical mobility, emotional reactions, social isolation and sleep, although there was no difference with regard to pain. Patients who were independent in activities of daily living had significantly better HRQOL as assessed by these scales than patients who were dependent in these activities.

The SIP is a widely used measure of HRQOL which has received widespread acceptance mainly because of its clinical comprehensiveness and its emphasis on observable behaviour, instead of on the more subjective health perceptions that are used in the NHP and the SF-36. Evaluations of the clinimetric properties of the SIP in patients with different diseases, including stroke, have shown that the instrument is reliable and valid but that its length poses a major disadvantage in stroke populations, as it takes 30 minutes or longer to complete the 136 items. Because of this, the SIP will not be described in greater detail here, but a recently described Stroke-Adapted SIP is discussed below.

The EuroQol is a generic instrument for the measurement of HRQOL which provides a simple descriptive profile of health in five dimensions (mobility, self-care, social, pain and psychological dimensions), each with three levels.[55] The patients' health state can therefore be classified into one of 243 theoretically possible health states, each of which has been assigned a utility (i.e. value to the patient). These utilities were assigned by a group of stroke-free individuals, and therefore probably require further validation. The EuroQol also includes a visual analogue scale on which patients rate their own health between 0 and 100, thereby providing an overall numerical estimate of their HRQOL. The relative brevity and simplicity of the EuroQol questionnaire achieved a better response rate in stroke survivors than the SF-36 (66% vs. 60%, $P = 0.002$).[56] There were also substantially more forms returned with no missing data for the EuroQol than for the SF-36 (66% vs. 55%, $P < 0.0001$).[56]

The validity of the EuroQol was assessed in a series of 152 patients with stroke who were all visited by a study nurse.[47] A total of 92 patients were able to complete the EuroQol without help, whilst the remaining 60 patients could only be assessed by interview. The EuroQol was demonstrated to have good concurrent validity – patients who reported problems in the EuroQol also reported dysfunction in the standard instruments for that domain. The EuroQol had reasonable discriminant validity, as the responses enabled separation between patients with differing stroke syndromes and stroke severity. HRQOL was poorest in all domains for patients with total anterior circulation strokes, and best for patients with posterior circulation strokes. Outcomes were similar in patients with partial anterior circulation strokes and with lacunar strokes, consistent with epidemiological data which suggest that partial anterior circulation strokes and lacunar strokes have very similar prognoses. Discriminant validity was also assessed in patients according to baseline stroke severity and, with the exception of the psychological functioning domain, better predicted prognosis was associated with better reported health status at follow-up. The EuroQol therefore appears to have acceptable concurrent and discriminant validity for the measurement of HRQOL after stroke.

The test–retest reliability of the EuroQol and SF-36 questionnaires has been assessed in a group of stroke patients who were taking part in the International Stroke Trial (IST).[57] Test–retest reliability was assessed using agreement statistics – weighted kappa statistics for the categorical domains of the EuroQol, and intra-class correlation coefficients for the EuroQol visual analogue scale, utility scores and SF-36. For the five categorical domains of the EuroQol, reproducibility was generally good, with kappa ranging from 0.63 to 0.80. The reproducibility of the domains of the SF-36 was qualitatively similar for all of the domains except mental health (the intra-class correlation coefficient was 0.28). However, the standard deviations of the differences in scores between test and retest were substantial (approximately ±20) for most domains, and were even larger for the physical and emotional role functioning domains. This degree of variability suggests that neither instrument would be suitable for serial studies within the same stroke patient, or for making serial comparisons between individual patients after stroke, unless very large differences over time were expected. Finally, for both instruments, reproducibility was better when the patient completed the questionnaires than when a proxy did so.

The Health Utilities Index (HUI) is based on concepts of functional capacity rather than on performance, and in addition to providing descriptive information on each of the attributes in the questionnaire, it is designed to produce a single summary measure of HRQOL. The HUI has been assessed in 74 patients who had suffered an ischaemic stroke within the last three months and in 37 family caregivers.[48] Inter-rater reliability was measured by evaluating the level of agreement between the patient and caregiver responses. In most instances the inter-rater reliability was acceptable, with values suggesting moderate to high agreement, and the kappa statistics ranging from 0.37 to 0.80. The lowest level of agreement was found for the distant vision question, perhaps because this ability is not discussed much between patients and caregivers. These data suggest that family caregivers can complete the HUI reliably when patients are unable to do so. Dorman *et al.* reached a similar conclusion using the EuroQol, finding moderate agreement between responses by patients and those by their proxies for the more directly observable domains of the EuroQol.[58] The level of agreement was only modest for the pain and social functioning domains, and no better than would be expected by chance for the psychological functioning domain (kappa = 0.05, 95% confidence interval = 0–0.43).

In summary, the generic measures of HRQOL which have attracted the most research interest are the EuroQol and the SF-36. Both of these have acceptable and qualitatively similar test–retest reliability when administered after stroke and completed by patients or their proxies.

Development and application of disease-specific measures

To date, work in this area of stroke disease has been very limited. The current literature contains only two measures which have been specifically developed for stroke patients, one being a stroke-adapted 30-item version of the Sickness Impact Profile (SA-SIP30)[59] and the other being a recently described Stroke-Specific Quality of Life Scale (SS-QOL).[60] The original SIP version usually takes 30 minutes or longer to complete, so a short stroke-adapted 30-item SIP version, the SA-SIP30, was constructed. The 12 subscales and 136 items of the original SIP were reduced to 8 subscales with 30 items on the basis of their relevance and homogeneity. This short-form version of the SIP was found to have high levels of internal reliability. Furthermore, principal-components analysis revealed the same two dimensions as in the original SIP (a physical and a psychosocial dimension). The SA-SIP30 explained 91% of the variation in scores of the original SIP in the same cohort of patients. External validity was estimated by comparing the scores of the SA-SIP30 with the original scores on the 136-item SIP for 88 patients from a different stroke study population. The Spearman rank correlation coefficient between the SA-SIP30 and the original SIP total scores was 0.96 ($P < 0.01$). However, this study only included patients who had normal communication skills, and it has not been tested in proxy respondents. Furthermore, there have been no tests of the responsiveness of the SA-SIP30. Studies of the responsiveness of the original SIP are also scarce, and the results are contradictory.

The domains and items of the SS-QOL were developed from patient interviews, and the items were then pilot-tested in patients one to three months after ischaemic stroke.[60] A total of 72 patients were enrolled in the study, with a mean age of 61 years. In total, 12 unidimensional domains were identified (mobility, energy, upper extremity function, work/productivity, mood, self-care, social roles, family roles, vision, language, thinking and personality). All of these domains demonstrated excellent internal reliability (Cronbach's alpha for each domain was greater than or equal to 0.73). Most domains were moderately correlated with similar domains of established outcome measures such as the SF-36 and NIHSS, with r^2 ranging from 0.3 to 0.5. The SS-QOL demonstrated moderate responsiveness to change between one and three months after stroke, with standardised effect sizes greater than 0.4. The mood and personality domains were noticeably less responsive across all instruments.

The disease-specific SS-QOL and the generic SF-36 were recently used to evaluate 71 patients one month after ischaemic stroke.[61] Stroke impairment and functional impairment were measured, as were symptoms of depression. A single question about overall HRQOL was used as the dependent variable. Using multivariate modelling, the authors found that variables associated with better overall HRQOL were higher (i.e. better) SS-QOL and Barthel Index scores, and lower (i.e. better) NIH Stroke Scale and Beck Depression Inventory scores. The SS-QOL score was an independent predictor of good overall HRQOL (odds ratio (OR) = 2.97; 95% CI = 1.3, 7.1; P = 0.01), as was the NIH Stroke Scale score (OR = 0.69; 95% CI = 0.47, 0.99; P = 0.05). The SF-36 scores were not associated with overall HRQOL ratings, suggesting that the disease-specific SS-QOL was more sensitive to meaningful changes in post-stroke patients than was the generic measure.

The preliminary results for reliability, content and construct validity and responsiveness of the SS-QOL are encouraging, but the issues of proxy respondents and interviewer vs. self-administration have not yet been addressed. Further validation of the SS-QOL in a larger sample that includes patients with more severe stroke is now in progress.

Conclusions

Stroke is the leading cause of adult disability, and the third commonest cause of death in the industrialised world. Despite the enormous personal, financial and social impact of stroke, the best method for assessing outcome remains unclear. It is critical to measure outcomes that are both relevant and important to stroke patients, particularly when examining the efficacy of new interventions. Commonly used stroke outcome measures tend to focus on physical impairment or the resultant disability, and other domains such as cognitive, language, psychological and social functioning skills have tended to be neglected.

An explosion of research into interventions in stroke has spawned a rapidly growing interest in the measurement of patient-centred outcomes. However, even in patients with an apparently good neurological recovery, HRQOL may not be restored to the presumed pre-stroke level. Assessment of HRQOL is particularly difficult after stroke, in which patients not only display diverse symptoms and signs, but also frequently experience language and communication difficulties. Indeed, recent studies suggest that scores for physical impairment correlate poorly with scores for language and cognitive impairment.

Generic HRQOL measures are much more widely used after stroke than are stroke-specific measures. The EuroQol and the SF-36 appear to be valid and reliable generic measures, with the largest evidence base to support their validity in stroke patients. Experience with disease-specific measures is currently very limited, but preliminary results obtained from the recently developed SS-QOL are encouraging.

References

1   Hatona S (1976) Experience from a multicentre stroke register: a preliminary report. *Bull WHO*. **54**: 541–53.
2   Martin J, Meltzer H and Elliott D (1988) *The Prevalence of Disability Among Adults*. HMSO, London.
3   Wolfe C (1996) The burden of stroke. In: C Wolfe, T Rudd and R Beech (eds) *Stroke Services and Research*. The Stroke Association, London.
4   Office of Population Censuses and Surveys (1995) *Mortality, Statistics, Causes. England and Wales 1992*. HMSO, London.
5   Wade D (1994) Stroke (acute cerebrovascular disease). In: A Stephens and J Raftery (eds) *Health Care Needs Assessments. Volume 1*. Radcliffe Medical Press, Oxford.
6   Bonita R (1992) Epidemiology of stroke. *Lancet*. **339**: 342–4.
7   Lalmgren R, Bamford J, Warlow C and Sandicock P (1987) Geographical and secular trends in stroke incidence. *Lancet*. **ii**: 1196–200.

8 Bamford J, Sandicock P, Dennis M and Warlow C (1990) A prospective study of acute cerebrovascular disease in the community: the Oxfordshire Community Stroke Project. Incidence, case fatality rates and overall outcome at one year after cerebral infarction, primary intracerebral and subarachnoid haemorrhage. *J Neurol Neurosurg Psychiatry*. **53**: 16–22.

9 Dennis MS, Burn JPS, Sandercock AG, Bamford JM, Wade DT and Warlow CP (1993) Long-term survival after first-ever stroke: the Oxfordshire Community Stroke Project. *Stroke*. **24**: 796–800.

10 Weddell JM and Beresford SSA (1979) *Planning for Stroke Patients. A Four-Year Descriptive Study of Home and Hospital Care*. HMSO, London.

11 Allen CMC (1983) Clinical diagnosis of the acute stroke syndrome. *Q J Med*. **208**: 515–23.

12 Sandercock P, Molyneux A and Warlow C (1995) Value of computed tomography in patients with stroke: the Oxfordshire Community Stroke Project. *BMJ*. **290**: 193–7.

13 Walker AE, Robins M and Weinfeld FD (1981) The National Survey of Stroke. *Stroke*. **12**(2) Suppl **1**: I13–I144.

14 Aho K, Harmsen P, Hatano S, Marquardsen J, Smnirnov E and Stisser T (1980) Cerebrovascular disease in the community: results of a WHO collaborative study. *Bull WHO*. **58**: 113–30.

15 Gordon C, Langton Hewer R and Wade DT (1987) Dysphagia in acute stroke. *BMJ*. **295**: 411–14.

16 Kidd D, Lawson J, Nesbitt R and MacMahon J (1993) Aspiration in acute stroke: a clinical study with videofluroscopy. *Q J Med*. **86**: 825–9.

17 Kumral E, Bogousslavsky J, Van Melle G, Regli F and Pierre P (1995) Headache at stroke onset: the Lausanne Stroke Registry. *J Neurol Neurosurg Psychiatry*. **58**: 490–2.

18 Burn J, Dennis M, Bamford J, Sandercock P, Wade D and Warlow C (1997) Epileptic seizures after a first stroke: the Oxfordshire Community Stroke Project. *BMJ*. **315**: 1582–7.

19 Scottish Intercollegiate Guidelines Network (1997) *Management of Patients with Stroke. 1. Assessment, Investigation, Immediate Management and Secondary Prevention.* Scottish Intercollegiate Guidelines Network, Edinburgh.

20 Hankey GH and Warlow CP (1999) Treatment and secondary prevention of stroke: evidence, costs and effects on individuals and populations. *Lancet.* **354**: 1457–63.

21 Langhorne P, Williams BO, Gilchrist W and Howie K (1993) Do stroke units save lives? *Lancet.* **342**: 395–8.

22 Aboderin I and Venables G (1996) Stroke management in Europe. *J Intern Med.* **240**: 173–80.

23 Chen ZM and Sandercock PAG (1999) Abstract. Indications for early aspirin use in acute ischaemic stroke: a combined analysis of over 40 000 randomised patients. *Stroke.* **30**: 243.

24 Wardlaw JM, Yamaguchi T and del Zoppo G (1999) Thrombolytic therapy versus control in acute ischaemic stroke (Cochrane Review). In: *The Cochrane Library.* Update Software, Oxford.

25 Individual Data Analysis of Antihypertensive Intervention Trials (INDIANA) Project Collaborators (1997) Effect of anti-hypertensive treatment in patients having already suffered from stroke: gathering the evidence. *Stroke.* **28**: 2557–62.

26 Hankey GJ (1999) Smoking and risk of stroke. *J Cardiovasc Risk.* **5**: 207–11.

27 Antiplatelet Trialist Collaboration (1994) Collaborative overview of randomised trials of antiplatelet therapy. 1. Prevention of death, myocardial infarction and stroke by prolonged antiplatelet therapy in various categories of patients. *BMJ.* **308**: 81–106.

28 Koudstaal P (1999) Secondary prevention following stroke or TIA in patients with non-rheumatic atrial fibrillation: anticoagulation therapy versus control (Cochrane Review). In: *The Cochrane Library.* Update Software, Oxford.

29 European Carotid Surgery Trialist Collaborative Group (1998) Randomised trial of endarterectomy for recently symptomatic carotid stenosis: the final results of the MRC European Carotid Surgery Trial (ECST). *Lancet.* **351**: 1379–87.

30 Bamford JM (1988) The classification and natural history of acute cerebrovascular disease. MD thesis, University of Manchester, Manchester.

31 Alan CMC (1994) Predicting the outcome of acute stroke: a prognostic score. *J Neurol Neurosurg Psychiatry.* **47**: 457–80.

32 Poungvarin N, Viriyavejaku IA and Komontri C (1991) Siriraj Stroke Score and validation study to distinguish supra-tentorial intracerebral haemorrhage from infarction. *BMJ.* **302**: 1565–7.

33 Parker VM, Wade DT and Langton Hewer R (1986) Loss of arm function after stroke: measurement, frequency and recovery. *Int Rehabil Med.* **8**: 69–73.

34 Wade DT and Colin C (1988) The Barthel ADL Index: a standard measure of physical disability? *Int Disabil Stud.* **10**: 64–7.

35 Rankin J (1957) Cerebral vascular accidents in patients over the age of 60. 2. Prognosis. *Scott Med J.* **2**: 200–15.

36 Van Swieten JC, Koudstaal PJ, Visser MC, Schouten AJA and Van Gijn J (1988) Inter-observer agreement for the assessment of handicap in stroke patients. *Stroke.* **19**: 604–7.

37 Orgogozo JM and Dartigues JF (1991) Methodology of clinical trials in acute cerebral ischaemia. *Cerebrovasc Dis.* **1**: 100–11.

38 Brott T, Adams HP, Olinger CP *et al.* (1989) Measurements of acute cerebral infarction: a clinical examination scale. *Stroke.* **20**: 864–70.

39 Adams RJ, Meador KJ, Sethi KD, Grotta JC and Thompson DS (1997) Graded neurological scale for use in acute hemispheric stroke treatment protocol. *Stroke.* **18**: 665–9.

40 Hantson L, De Weerdt W, De Keyser J *et al.* (1994) The European Stroke Scale. *Stroke.* **25**: 2215–19.

41 Scandinavian Stroke Study Group (1985) Multicentre trial of haemodilution in ischaemic stroke: background and study protocol. *Stroke.* **16**: 885–90.

42 Guyatt GH, Feeny DH and Patrick DL (1993) Measuring health-related quality of life. *Ann Intern Med.* **118**: 622–9.

43 Ebrahim S, Barer D and Nouri F (1996) Use of the Nottingham Health Profile with patients after a stroke. *J Epidemiol Commun Health.* **40**: 166–9.

44 De Bruin AF, De Witte LP, Stevens FCJ and Diederiksj JPM (1992) Sickness Impact Profile: the state of the art of a generic functional status measure. *Soc Sci Med.* **35**: 1008–14.

45 Anderson C, Laubscher S and Burns R (1996) Validation of the Short-Form 36 (SF-36) Health Survey Questionnaire among stroke patients. *Stroke.* **27**: 1812–16.

46 Pickard AS, Johnson JA, Penn A, Lau F and Noseworthy T (1999) Replicability of SF-36 summary scores by the SF-12 in stroke patients. *Stroke.* **30**: 1213–17.

47 Dorman PJ, Waddell F, Slattery J, Dennis M and Sander-cock P (1997) Is the EuroQol a valid measure of health-related quality of life after stroke? *Stroke.* **28**: 1876–82.

48 Mathis SD, Bates MM, Pasta DJ, Cisternas MG, Feeny D and Patrick DL (1997) Use of the Health Utilities Index with stroke patients and their caregivers. *Stroke.* **28**: 1888–94.

49 Kaplan RM, Anderson JP and Ganiats TG (1993) The Quality of Well-Being Scale: a rationale for a single quality-of-life index. In: SR Walker and RM Rosser (eds) *Quality of Life Assessment: Key Issues in the 1990s.* Kluwer Academic Publishers, Dordrecht.

50 Ware J and Sherbourne C (1992) The Moss 36-item Short-Form health survey. 1. Conceptual framework and item selection. *Med Care.* **30**: 473–83.

51 Brazier JE, Harper R, Jones NMB *et al.* (1992) Validating the SF-36 Health Survey Questionnaire: new outcome measure for primary care. *BMJ.* **305**: 160–64.

52 Jenkinson C, Coulter A and Wright L (1993) The SF-36 Health Survey Questionnaire: normative data from a large random sample of working age adults. *BMJ*. **306**: 1437–40.

53 Ware JE, Kosinski M and Keller SD (1996) A 12-item Short-Form health survey: construction of scales and preliminary test of reliability and validity. *Med Care*. **34**: 220–26.

54 Indredavik B, Bakke F, Slørdahl SA, Rokseth R and Haheim LL (1998). Stroke unit treatment improves long-term quality of life. A randomised controlled trial. *Stroke*. **29**: 895–9.

55 The EuroQol Group (1990) EuroQol – a new facility for the measurement of health-related quality of life. *Health Policy*. **16**: 199–208.

56 Dorman P, Slattery J, Farrell B, Dennis M and Sandercock P (1997) A randomised comparison of the EuroQol and Short-Form 36 after stroke. *BMJ*. **315**: 461.

57 Dorman P, Slattery J, Farrell B, Denis M and Sandercock P for the United Kingdom Collaborators in the International Stroke Trial (IST) (1998) Qualitative comparison of the reliability of health status assessments with the EuroQol and SF-36 questionnaires after stroke. *Stroke*. **29**: 63–8.

58 Dorman PJ, Waddle F, Slattery J, Denis M and Sandercock P (1997) Are proxy assessments of health status after stroke with the EuroQol questionnaire feasible, accurate and unbiased? *Stroke*. **28**: 1883-7.

59 Van Straten A, De Haan RJ, Limberg M, Schuling J, Bossuit PM, Van de Bos GAM (1997) A stroke adapted 30-item version of the Sickness Impact Profile to assess quality of life (SA-SIP30). *Stroke*. **28**: 2155–61.

60 Williams LS, Weinberger M, Harris LE, Clark DO and Biller J (1999) Development of a Stroke-Specific Quality-of-Life Scale. *Stroke*. **30**: 1362–9.

61 Williams LS, Weinberger M, Harris LE and Biller JB (1999) Measuring quality of life in a way that is meaningful to stroke patients. *Neurology*. **53**: 1839–43.

6
Epilepsy

Ann Jacoby, Gus A Baker and
David Chadwick

Introduction

Over the last two decades, interest in documenting the quality of life of people with epilepsy has moved from what Scambler[1] has described as 'pre-formal studies' to its formal quantification as an indicator of health outcome.[2,3] Hermann[4] has proposed that any attempt at quantifying quality of life in relation to epilepsy must adopt a broad vision of the term, since the nature of the condition is such that any assessment must encompass both 'within-the-skin' and 'beyond-the-skin' variables. Hermann's list of essential domains for quality-of-life assessments in epilepsy covers symptoms, functional status, social functioning, sleep and rest, energy, health perceptions, general life satisfaction, role activities, emotional state and cognition. His view is supported by empirical investigations,[5-7] which have identified a wide range of quality-of-life concerns among people with epilepsy. In this chapter we shall describe the quality-of-life measures currently available for epilepsy, and give examples of their application as measures of outcome. However, in order to contextualise our discussion, we shall begin with a brief examination of the key clinical considerations and the significance of a diagnosis of epilepsy from a social scientific perspective, since both have an important bearing on its impact on quality of life.

Epilepsy as a clinical condition

Epilepsy is a common neurological disorder that ranges in expression from a small number of self-limiting seizures to long-term, frequent seizures which are treatment resistant. Epidemiological studies are reasonably consistent in their estimates of the incidence and prevalence of epilepsy,[8] the age-related incidence being around 20–70 per 100 000 and the prevalence 4–10 per 1000.[9] It is estimated that around 50 million people have epilepsy world-wide, with around 400 000 individuals in the UK.

Epilepsy is no longer viewed as a single disease entity but as a group of disorders in which seizures occur. The current classification of epilepsy syndromes[10] divides epilepsy into the symptomatic epilepsies, that is those with a recognisable cause, and the idiopathic or crytogenic epilepsies, without an obvious cause. In the majority of cases, no identifiable cause for epilepsy can be found, although with developments in brain-imaging techniques this picture is likely to change. Seizures themselves take a variety of forms, but are broadly classifiable into partial seizures (those whose onset is localised to one side of the brain) and generalised seizures (where there is no evidence of local onset).[11] Another fundamental division is between seizures in which the affected person's consciousness is impaired, and those in which it remains unaffected.[12]

From community-based studies it is now clear that in about 70–80% of people with epilepsy their condition is benign and they will enter remission soon after commencing anticonvulsant treatment. In the remaining 20–30% of cases, seizures will prove unresponsive to therapy, and in the most severe cases the epilepsy may be accompanied by learning disabilities. A number of factors have been identified as influencing the prognosis of epilepsy,[13] the most important of these being aetiology, seizure type and the presence of an abnormal EEG.

Currently, anticonvulsant drugs represent the major treatment approach for epilepsy. Treatment policies are variable, but in the UK people who have had only one seizure are not generally classified as having epilepsy. Treatment is generally considered to be indicated when two or more unprovoked seizures occur relatively close together.[9] The current convention of choosing particular drugs for particular seizure types and epilepsy syndromes is not always fully supported by evidence, but there is general agreement that carbamazepine and sodium valproate should be used as first-line therapies. Their dominance may be challenged by the newer anti-epileptics as information about their relative efficacy, tolerability and cost-effectiveness becomes available.

A major consideration governing the choice between currently licensed anti-epileptic drugs (AEDs) is their relative toxicity, which can be acute and dose related, acute and idiosyncratic, or chronic.[9] All anti-epileptics have adverse effects on cognitive function, even at therapeutic concentrations, most are neurotoxic, and all of those that have been sufficiently thoroughly investigated have also been shown to be associated with other much rarer but serious complications in very small numbers of patients. Because these drugs are associated with unwanted side-effects, patients with epilepsy are faced with the decision of whether or not to withdraw from treatment once they have achieved remission of their seizures. The largest study to examine the outcomes of anti-epileptic drug withdrawal was the UK MRC Anti-epileptic Drug Withdrawal Study,[14] which showed that, in individuals whose epilepsy was in remission, the risk of relapse was substantial under a policy of withdrawal when compared to one of continued treatment, especially during the first year. This may be because drug withdrawal recipitates seizure recurrence in patients who would be at risk of further seizures regardless of the treatment policy. Interestingly, the study found no substantial differences in psychosocial outcomes in relation to treatment policy, which suggests that for some patients at least the benefits of achieving good seizure control by taking AEDs are outweighed by the costs of their side-effects.[15]

Epilepsy as a social label

Historically, epilepsy was a condition with extremely negative connotations, and one which was consequently highly stigmatising.[16] Even today stigma remains a defining feature of epilepsy for many of the people who are affected by it. Since even for the large majority whose condition remits it can never be said with absolute certainty that their epilepsy is 'cured', they may continue to face both statutory limitations and discrimination over their condition long after their seizures have been clinically controlled. Although legislation such as the UK Disability Discrimination Act (1995) and the US Americans with Disabilities Act (1990) seeks to protect people with chronic conditions, including epilepsy, from prejudice and unfair discrimination, and research shows that public attitudes to epilepsy have improved over time,[17,18] there is still plenty of evidence that people with epilepsy continue to be concerned about the possibility of being treated differently because of their condition.[19–24] It appears that, for many of them, the stigma of epilepsy is still 'serious and real',[25] and continues to have the potential to limit their social and psychological functioning and hence their broader quality of life.

The measurement of quality of life in epilepsy

Available measures

To date, the main approaches to quality-of-life assessment in epilepsy have been fourfold, namely those which have involved the development of a novel quality-of-life measure, such as the WPSI[6] (see below) or the Social Effects Scale,[5] those that involve the use of a previously developed generic profile with customised additions, such as the Epilepsy Surgery Inventory[26] or the QOLIE[27] (see p. 101), those that utilise a battery of previously validated scales addressing specific quality-of-life domains together with additional disease-specific items, such as the Liverpool Quality-of-Life Battery,[28] and those that espouse the patient-generated approach.[29]

Washington Psychosocial Seizure Inventory (WPSI)

The oldest and probably most widely used epilepsy-specific measure that formally addresses quality-of-life issues is the Washington Psychosocial Seizure Inventory (WPSI).[30] Developed in the 1970s to evaluate the psychosocial problems commonly seen in adults with seizure disorders, it consists of 132 items across eight scales, namely family background, emotional adjustment, interpersonal adjustment, vocational adjustment, financial status, adjustment to seizures, medicines and medical management and overall psychosocial functioning. The WPSI was intended as a comprehensive, systematic and *objective* assessment of psychosocial problems, this emphasis on its objectivity being in marked contrast to the more recent emphasis on the importance of subjective assessment. High levels of internal consistency and test–retest reliability have been reported for the WPSI, and criterion validity is supported by correlations between WPSI scale scores and professional ratings. The WPSI has been criticised for its dichotomous response format, the fact that scale composition rests solely on statistical grounds, and the fact that because it is specific for epilepsy, it does not allow comparisons with other non-epilepsy populations.[26] Recently, its authors have acknowledged its limitations in relation to current concepts of quality of life, in response to which they have developed a WPSI quality-of-life scale,[31] consisting of 36 items from the original.

The Epilepsy Social Effects Scale (ESES)

The ESES was designed to investigate the social effects of their condition on adults with epilepsy of varying duration and

Table 6.1: Areas of psychosocial function covered by the Epilepsy Social Effects Scale (ESES)

A1	Acceptance of the diagnosis
A2	Fear of having seizures
A3	Fear of stigma affecting employment
A4	Lack of confidence about the future
A5	Lack of confidence about travelling
A6	Adverse effects on social life
A7	Adverse effects on leisure pursuits
A8	Change of outlook on life/self
A9	Difficulty with the family
A10	Attitude to taking medication
A11	Attitude to the medical profession
A12	Depression or emotional reactions
A13	Feelings of increased isolation
A14	Lack of energy/lethargy

Reproduced from Chaplin et al.[5] with permission.

severity.[5] A large pool of statements about the impact of epilepsy was generated through in-depth interviews with patients. Both patients and physicians were then asked to group the statements into distinct areas, and additional areas were generated from a search of the relevant literature. In total, 21 areas of psychosocial adjustment were identified but, following a criterion-related validity study, only 14 areas were included in the final version of the scale. Among the areas covered are attitude towards epilepsy and seizures, fear of stigma, concern about personal and social relationships, lack of confidence in performing particular activities, problems with healthcare and medications, emotional problems and social isolation (see Table 6.1).

Epilepsy Surgery Inventory (ESI-55)

The generic health status measure, the SF-36,[32] is the basis of two recent quality-of-life measurement initiatives in epilepsy.

Vickrey *et al.*[26] elected to use it as the stem for their Epilepsy Surgery Inventory (ESI-55), supplementing it with additional items which tap aspects of quality of life that are identified as being of particular relevance to epilepsy patients. To the items present in the SF-36, the authors added five items relating to cognitive function, eight items relating to role limitations, four items relating to health perceptions and two items relating to overall quality of life. The final scale includes subscales to assess health perceptions, energy and fatigue, overall quality of life, social function, emotional well-being, cognitive function, physical function, pain, and role limitations due to physical, emotional and memory problems. The reliability of the ESI-55 is good (with alpha coefficients ranging from 0.68 to 0.88), multi-trait scaling analyses support item discrimination across the scales, and factor analysis has confirmed previously identified mental and physical health factors and a third factor defined by cognitive function and role limitation scales. Finally, construct validity was supported by correlations between ESI-55 scale scores and a mood profile scale, and by the finding that the scores of patients who were seizure-free following epilepsy surgery were better than those of patients who continued to have seizures or auras.

Quality of Life in Epilepsy (QOLIE) scales

The SF-36 is also the basis of the series of scales developed by the QOLIE Development Group,[27] referred to as the QOLIE-89 (17 scales and 89 items), the QOLIE-31 (7 scales and 31 items) and the QOLIE-10 (10 items selected from the 7 QOLIE-31 scales). These scales are intended for broader application than the surgery-specific one developed by Vickrey. The domains covered by the two longer versions of the scale are shown in Table 6.2. Factor analysis of the 17 scales in the QOLIE-89 revealed four dimensions, namely epilepsy-targeted, cognitive, mental health and physical health. Devinsky *et al.*[27] have

Table 6.2: Domains of the Quality of Life in Epilepsy (QOLIE-89) instrument

Health perceptions	Memory
Seizure worry*	Language
Physical function	Medication effects*
Role limitation – physical	Social support
Role limitation – emotional	Social function*
Pain	Social isolation
Overall quality of life*	Health discouragement
Emotional well-being*	Sexual function
Energy/fatigue*	Overall health*
Attention/concentration*	

*The QOLIE-31 includes items taken from these scales. Reproduced from Cramer[78] with permission.

provided cross-sectional data from 304 adult patients attending 25 US epilepsy centres to support the reliability and construct validity of the measure in its long form. Patients' scores on the QOLIE-89 were significantly correlated with their scores on the Profile of Mood States. Their scores were negatively correlated with high seizure frequency, scores on a systemic and neurological toxicity scale and with health care utilisation. They were positively correlated with higher levels of education and being in employment. The authors of the QOLIE scales regard them as serving somewhat different purposes, with the two longer scales being intended for research and the 10-item version serving as a useful screening tool for clinical practice.

The Subjective Handicap of Epilepsy (SHE) scale

Justification for the SHE scale[33] is derived from the World Health Organisation conceptualisation that the consequences of disease occur at the level of impairment, disability and handicap.

The scale contains 32 items in 6 subscales, namely work and activities (8 items), social and personal (4 items), self-perception (5 items), physical (4 items), life satisfaction (4 items) and a change scale (7 items).

The construct validity of the SHE was supported by the finding that scale scores were responsive to the effects of increasing seizure frequency and outcome after epilepsy surgery. The internal consistency of the scales ranged from 0.8 to 0.9 (Cronbach's alpha), and the test–tetest reliability was also satisfactory. The authors of the SHE present their scale as a response to the technical and conceptual difficulties surrounding quality-of-life measurement, and suggest that it is potentially more useful than the traditional approach adopted by other epilepsy quality-of-life researchers.

The Liverpool Quality-of-Life Battery for Epilepsy

The Liverpool Quality-of-Life Battery addresses aspects of physical, social and psychological functioning, employing both previously validated and novel multi-item scales to assess seizure severity, symptoms and general health, social activities, support and limitations, employment status and limitations, driving, feelings of stigma, anxiety and depression, self-esteem and sense of mastery. The starting point for development of the battery was a UK Medical Research Council-funded randomised clinical trial of anti-epileptic drug withdrawal,[15] and it was subsequently refined for application in clinical trials of novel anti-epileptics.[34] The Liverpool battery is model driven,[35] and allows different combinations of domain-specific scales to be selected, depending on the particular research question under consideration (*see* Table 6.3). Although not all of the scales in the model were originally developed for epilepsy, all of them were validated in subjects with epilepsy before being incorporated. The most widely applied novel scale in the

Table 6.3: Liverpool Quality-of-Life Assessment Battery for Epilepsy

Scale	Number of items
Seizure Severity Scale[36]	20
Nottingham Health Profile[79]	38
Hospital Anxiety and Depression Scale[80]	14
Affect Balance Scale[81]	10
Self-Esteem Scale[82]	10
Mastery Scale[54]	7
Stigma Scale[23]	3
Life Fulfilment Scale[38]	26
Impact of Epilepsy Scale[37]	10
Adverse Drug Effects Profile[39]	19

Liverpool battery is the Seizure Severity Scale,[36] which has been used in a number of clinical trials of novel anti-epileptic drugs. Other measures developed by the group include scales to assess patient-perceived impact of epilepsy on daily functioning,[37] feelings of stigma associated with epilepsy,[23] life fulfilment,[38] and adverse drug effects.[39] The scales in the battery have been shown to have clinical validity with regard to seizure frequency and epilepsy severity. There is also some evidence of their responsiveness.[34]

Side-Effect and Life Satisfaction Scale (SEALS)[40]

A rather more limited measure of quality of life in epilepsy is provided by the SEALS Inventory, which its authors claim fills a need, particularly in the context of clinical trials, for 'a more compact, more behaviourally orientated scale' than those already discussed. The SEALS is a 50-item self-report questionnaire developed by Brown and Tomlinson[41] and standardised by Gilham et al.[40] Principal-components analysis at the stage of its initial development suggested an underlying scale structure of five factors. Five factors were also produced in the later validation study by Gilham et al., but they do not match the original five, being identified in this second analysis as 'cognition', 'dysphoria', 'temper', 'tiredness' and 'worry'. Further work is needed to confirm that it is reasonable to adopt the more recent structure. The SEALS appears to be clinically sensitive, with patients experiencing chronic intractable seizures having significantly poorer scores than those who were newly diagnosed on two of the five factors (cognition and dysphoria) and better scores on one of them (worry).

Two other patient group-specific measures are worth mentioning briefly here. The Quality of Life in Newly Diagnosed Epilepsy Patients Assessment (NEWQOL)[42] is a 93-item self-administered battery consisting of 8 multi-item scales measuring anxiety and depression, social activities, symptoms, locus of control, neuropsychological problems, stigma, work limitations and epilepsy worry. An initial psychometric validation study showed that the scales had high discriminant validity, good test–retest reliability and internal consistency. Their validity was supported by the finding that scores varied according to seizure frequency and patient-assessed severity. The NEWQOL is currently being used in a number of studies, but results are not yet available. The Epilepsy and Learning Disability Quality of Life Questionnaire (ELDQOL)[43] was developed from first principles for use in patients with epilepsy accompanied by learning disability. The ELDQOL consists of a 66-item instrument, with subscales to assess seizure severity (14 items), drug-related side-effects (18 items), mood (14 items) and behaviour (9 items), as well as single items relating to experience of seizure-related injuries, health and quality of life overall. The measure is designed for completion by a proxy, in this instance a parent or other informal carer. The instrument has good content and construct validity, is reliable (alpha coefficients range from 0.71

to 0.84 and test–retest scores range from 0.67 to 0.84) and appears to be acceptable. There is also some evidence from a recent randomised study of its responsiveness to change.[44]

A patient-elicited approach to quality-of-life assessment

In the field of epilepsy, this approach has been the focus of the work by Trimble et al.,[29,45] who used the repertory-grid technique to determine within five core areas (physical, cognitive, social, psychological and work/economic) what specific aspects of functioning are important to individual patients. Within this framework, subjects then design their own Quality-of-Life Assessment Schedule (QOLAS), rating the degree to which each aspect they have identified is currently problematic. In the original QOLAS interview, they were also asked to rate other situations and individuals, in order to construct a 'grid' of their view of their current situation in relation to their past, their expectations for the future and other people. Since this version was found to be rather lengthy and cumbersome, attempts have subsequently been made to streamline the interview and its scoring.[45,46] The reliability, validity and specificity of the original QOLAS were thoroughly investigated by Kendrick,[47] and testing of the simplified QOLAS-R is currently in progress.

As is apparent from this review, there is now a large number of potential quality-of-life measures from which the epilepsy researcher can choose. A sentiment with which we have some sympathy is that expressed by Hays,[48] who commented that future research efforts in relation to adults with epilepsy might most profitably be applied to further evaluation of those measures that are already available, rather than to reinventing the quality-of-life assessment wheel. In the next section, the methodological considerations that are applicable to quality-of-life assessment generally will be briefly considered in relation to assessments in epilepsy.

Methodological issues

Generic vs. epilepsy-specific measures

Despite the received wisdom that condition-specific measures will be more responsive than generic measures, work by Langfitt[49] and Wiebe et al.[50] in relation to epilepsy suggests otherwise. Langfitt compared the psychometric properties of the WPSI, the ESI-55 and a generic health status measure, namely the Sickness Impact Profile (SIP).[51] He found that the WPSI had poorer face, content and criterion validity than either the ESI-55 or the SIP, and he concluded that because its focus is narrower, the WPSI provides a less valid description of the impact of epilepsy on quality of life than the other two measures. Wiebe et al.[50] compared the responsiveness of the WPSI to that of two other instruments, namely the ESI-55 and a 90-item symptom check-list intended to serve as a measure of psychological function and distress. All three instruments registered some degree of change, all of them changed in the same direction in the group of patients with a better seizure outcome, and when improvement was detected it was consistently larger in the group with better seizure outcome. However, the WPSI showed inferior responsiveness to both of the other scales, and it appeared to be relatively unresponsive to small and medium-size changes.

Furthermore, in their comparison Wiebe et al. found that, with one exception, none of the epilepsy-specific scales in the ESI-55 performed better than the SF-36 generic scales contained in it — and the exception was itself composed of seven generic items and only two epilepsy-specific items. Wiebe's finding parallels that of Guyatt et al.,[52] who reported that an age-specific instrument for frail elderly people did not show greater responsiveness than generic instruments.

The usefulness of combining generic and epilepsy-specific scales has also been examined by Wagner et al.[53] They administered a series of measures, including the SF-36, the Impact of

Epilepsy Scale, the Liverpool Seizure Severity Scale, a modified version of the Mastery scale[54] and a novel two-item Epilepsy Distress Scale in order to evaluate their practicality and psychometric properties. The quality of the data was high and, with few exceptions, both the generic and epilepsy-specific measures satisfied standard psychometric criteria, and were shown to be valid in relation to two clinical criteria, namely disease severity and symptoms. Epilepsy-specific scales were generally best at discriminating between groups of patients experiencing differing disease severity, and generic ones were most effective in differentiating between groups with differing experience of symptoms.

Battery, profile or index measures

As described above, approaches to quality-of-life measurement in epilepsy have included the use of both scale batteries and profile measures. Mindful of the potential value of an overall scale score for cost-utility studies, the authors of the ESI-55 have derived one by computing three composite scores – mental health, physical health and role function – and averaging them to obtain a summary score.[55] The theoretical minimum score on this overall scale is 0 (representing worst possible health) and the maximum is 100 (representing best possible health). Further work is required to calibrate the range of this overall score. Similarly, an overall score and four composite scores can be computed for the QOLIE-89 by weighting and summing individual scale scores.

Psychometric issues

Instruments developed to measure quality of life in epilepsy have been formally evaluated according to the basic psychometric principles of validity, reliability and responsiveness to varying degrees. Generally speaking, there is a good deal of evidence about their validity and reliability, and rather less about their responsiveness to change (*see* Table 6.4). It is also worth noting that test–retest reliability is largely confined to calculation of Pearson's *r*, rather than the preferred intra-class correlation coefficient.[56]

Use of proxy information

As in other neurological conditions, there will be situations where people with epilepsy are unable to respond themselves and researchers have to resort to obtaining proxy information from a relative, friend or formal carer. Hays *et al.*[57] compared responses to an epilepsy-specific quality-of-life measure, namely the QOLIE-89, of 292 people with epilepsy and their designated proxies, and reported only moderate correlations between the two with (not surprisingly) better agreement for directly observable measures of function than for the more subjective measures. Proxies reported better functioning on three scales of cognitive function than did patients, whereas patients reported more positive health perceptions and less seizure distress, and in some domains the lack of agreement was sufficiently large to introduce bias. Despite this, the authors conclude that, for group comparisons, proxy respondents can reasonably be substituted for patients themselves.

Interpretation of quality-of-life measures

Although the importance of the concept of the 'minimally important difference'[58,59] is highlighted by results from recent clinical trials of novel anti-epileptic treatments, this is an issue that has yet to be robustly addressed for epilepsy. Some relevant information will accrue over time as the results of studies enter the public domain and allow quality-of-life profiles

Table 6.4: Summary of available evidence of psychometric properties of quality-of-life measures for adults with epilepsy

Measure	Internal consistency	Reproducibility	Content validity	Construct validity	Responsiveness
WPSI	✓	✓	✓	✓	✓
Social Effects Scale	✓	✓	✓	✓	✗
ESI-55	✓	✗	✓	✓	✓
QOLIE-89	✓	✓	✓	✓	✗
Liverpool Battery					
Seizure severity	✓	✓	✓	✓	✓
Impact of epilepsy	✓	✓	✓	✓	✗
Mastery	✓	✓	✓	✓	✓
Self-esteem	✓	✗	✓	✓	✓
Affect balance	✓	✗	✓	✓	✓
HAD	✓	✗	✓	✓	✓
Stigma	✓	✗	✓	✓	✓
NHP	✓	✗	✓	✓	✓
Life fulfilment	✓	✗	✓	✓	✗
Adverse drug events	✓	✗	✓	✓	✗
SEALS	?	?	?	✓	✗
SHE	✓	✓	✓	✓	✗
NEWQOL	✓	✓	✓	✓	✗
ELDQOL	✓	✓	✓	✓	✓
Repertory Grid Assessment	*	✓	✓	✓	✓

*Not applicable owing to the nature of the assessment tool.

associated with particular clinical features of epilepsy or its treatment to be defined, but currently there is a dearth of methodological research activity to inform this. Wagner and Vickrey[60] have recently emphasised the need for clinically useful interpretation manuals for quality-of-life assessment, which display quality-of-life profiles of patients with differing epilepsy syndromes, seizure types and frequency, as well as differing treatments.

Cross-cultural issues

All of the currently available quality-of-life measures for epilepsy were developed in the UK or the USA, and so require cross-cultural validation if they are to be employed elsewhere. Given that many clinical trials in epilepsy are now international in focus, cross-cultural validation is being recognised as a basic requirement for their use, and a number of initiatives are under way, funded mainly by the pharmaceutical industry. For example, Rapp et al. have recently published an evaluation of the Liverpool battery in US patients,[61] and the Social Effects Scale has been translated into Swedish, where it is currently being used to assess the outcome of an epilepsy surgery programme. Issues relating to the translation and validation of questionnaires for use cross-culturally are discussed in Chapter 9 of this book.

Application of quality-of-life measures in epilepsy

Quality-of-life measures have been used to provide descriptive data about people with epilepsy and, more recently, as measures of outcome within the framework of clinical trials of the treatment of this disorder. It has been suggested that quality-of-life measures could also be employed in routine clinical practice, although as yet there is relatively little evidence of the utility of using structured questionnaires over clinicians' informal questioning. In this chapter, we focus attention on studies where quality-of-life instruments were used as measures of treatment outcome. Descriptive quality-of-life studies using formal quality-of-life instruments to which we would draw the reader's attention include those by Collings,[62] Jacoby,[63] Baker et al.[64] and Buck et al.[65]

To our knowledge, the first clinical trial in epilepsy to incorporate a systematic assessment of quality of life was not concerned with comparing different drugs for epilepsy, but with different management strategies. The UK MRC Anti-Epileptic Drug Withdrawal Study[15] aimed to answer the question of whether, in patients who achieve a remission of their seizures (defined as being seizure-free for at least two years), medication could reasonably be withdrawn. Patients were randomised to either slow withdrawal of their anti-epileptic medication or its continuation, and they were followed for a minimum of one year. The primary outcome for the study was the percentage of patients who remained seizure-free under the two treatment policies. By two years after randomisation, 41% of those in whom treatment was withdrawn had relapsed, compared to only 22% of those who remained on medication. Yet despite the substantial clinical risk, there was little evidence to support the hypothesis that this would be accompanied by a parallel increased risk in relation to quality of life. For all of the domains considered, the effect of drug withdrawal was small and non-significant, suggesting that for some patients the threat of seizures was counter-balanced by the threat of adverse drug effects.

The first trial of a novel anti-epileptic to employ such an approach examined the efficacy of lamotrigine as an add-on treatment in adults with intractable epilepsy.[34] A total of 61 subjects completed the Liverpool quality-of-life battery on entry to the trial and at the end of the treatment. Small but significant differences in patients' perceptions of the severity of their seizures were demonstrated between those who were on active treatment and those who were not. In addition, patients who were treated with lamotrigine reported significant improvements in affect balance and sense of mastery compared to those on placebo. Of the 61 patients who completed the study, 41 individuals elected to continue taking lamotrigine after the end of the trial, despite the fact that only 10 patients had achieved a more than 50% reduction in seizure frequency – the standard marker of efficacy in such trials. A comparison of those who opted to continue with those who did not revealed that the former had a significantly better psychological profile during the active phase of the trial (*see* Table 6.5), confirming anecdotal evidence of the mood-enhancing effect of the active compound and its ability to reduce seizure severity.

A limited quality-of-life evaluation was performed as part of a trial of another novel anti-epileptic, Gabapentin.[66] Adult patients with medically refractory partial seizures were randomised to one of three different dosing regimens (600, 1200 or 2400 mg/day), added initially to other anti-epileptic drug medication. Concurrent anti-epileptics were then tapered over a 10-week period, until Gabapentin monotherapy was achieved. Quality of life was assessed prior to randomisation and on exit from the study, the measures of adjustment including the Profile of Mood States, the WPSI and a visual analogue mood rating scale. Patients who were treated with Gabapentin showed statistically significant improvements in adjustment, independent of any reduction in seizure frequency, and more favourable changes were noted when two concurrent anti-epileptic drugs were discontinued, rather than one.

The SEALS Inventory has been used to evaluate lamotrigine and carbamazepine monotherapy in the treatment of 256 patients with newly diagnosed epilepsy.[40] The SEALS was completed at baseline and at subsequent assessment points during the double-blind study. For each of the five SEALS subscales, patients on lamotrigine showed a significantly greater change in a positive direction than those on carbamazepine, after controlling for baseline seizure frequency, change in seizure frequency, age and gender.

Table 6.5: HRQOL scores for patients continuing vs. those not continuing on lamotrigine

Variable	Continuing mean score (95% CIs)	Non-continuing mean score (95% CIs)	P-value
Seizure severity scale: percept	24.82 (23.47, 26.17)	25.68 (24.10, 27.26)	0.446
Seizure severity scale: ictal	18.50 (16.49, 20.51)	21.84 (19.13, 24.55)	0.061
NHP energy	0.71 (0.42, 1.00)	0.63 (0.20, 1.06)	0.765
NHP pain	0.79 (0.20, 1.38)	0.06 (0.00, 0.32)	0.148
NHP emotional reaction	1.63 (1.09, 2.18)	3.11 (1.96, 4.25)	0.012
NHP sleep	0.82 (0.39, 1.24)	1.05 (0.78, 1.68)	0.540
NHP social isolation	0.76 (0.39, 1.11)	1.47 (0.87, 2.08)	0.038
NHP physical mobility	1.26 (0.68, 1.85)	0.42 (0.15, 0.69)	0.066
Activities of daily living	43.97 (41.49, 46.45)	43.10 (39.79, 46.50)	0.691
Anxiety	5.76 (4.33, 7.20)	9.90 (7.78, 12.01)	0.002
Depression	3.87 (2.92, 4.81)	5.53 (4.05, 7.01)	0.060
Happiness	4.27 (2.85, 5.69)	1.69 (−0.67, 4.05)	0.057
Total mood disturbance	20.68 (13.52, 27.84)	37.11 (26.07, 48.15)	0.015
Self-esteem	30.57 (28.88, 32.26)	27.33 (24.81, 29.85)	0.039
Mastery	20.74 (19.59, 21.91)	17.65 (15.63, 19.66)	0.008

NHP, Nottingham Health Profile.

Quality-of-life outcomes in routine clinical practice

It has been suggested that a third possible use of quality-of-life measures is as a clinical tool within routine practice. Their use in this setting may improve the quality of care of epilepsy patients by increasing the rate of detection of their functional limitations and psychological distress, by allowing the patient and physician to decide jointly on appropriate quality-of-life outcomes and quantify progress towards their achievement, and by increasing patients' satisfaction with care and their own quality-of-life.[60] One brief quality-of-life measure recently recommended for routine use is the 10-item QOLIE,[67] which can be completed by a patient in several minutes and reviewed rapidly by the physician. The 10 items cover three distinct topics, namely medication effects, mental health and role functioning. Its authors argue that using short-form measures allows healthcare providers under pressure from limited resources to assess a variety of issues without the potentially costly input required for administration and scoring of longer instruments. However, it is salutary to note that Wagner et al.,[68] when they assessed the benefits of routine use of the SF-36 health survey in epilepsy care, reported that physicians rated it as moderately useful for communication in only 14% of consultations, and for patient management in only 8%. This raises the fundamental question of whether the acquisition of new information necessarily results in action.

Assessment of quality of life in children and adolescents with epilepsy

This review has focused on assessment of quality of life in adults with epilepsy. As is the case for other chronic conditions, considerably less has been done to measure quality of life in children with epilepsy, in part because the rapid developmental changes that occur during childhood make assessment of quality of life more complex than for adults. Historically, children — like older people — have been excluded from clinical trials of new treatments, so that one impetus to the development of quality-of-life scales for them has been missing. However, interest in developing such measures for children and adolescents with epilepsy is increasing, and we shall briefly touch on current work.

As part of a wider research programme to assess the factors that determine quality of life in children with epilepsy,[69,70] Austin's group in the USA has developed a number of scales, including the Child Attitude to Illness Scale (CATIS),[71] the Coping Health Inventory for Children (CHIC)[72] and the Child Concerns About Seizures Scale (JK Austin, personal communication). The first of these, the CATIS, was designed to measure children's feelings about having a chronic condition, and it consists of 17 items developed at a reading level appropriate for independent completion by children aged 8 to 12 years. It has been shown to have good internal consistency and test–retest reliability, and its construct validity is supported by confirmatory factor analysis. The CHIC is a 45-item measure intended for completion by parents and designed to address five coping patterns, namely competence and optimism, withdrawal, irritability/moodiness, compliance and support-seeking. The scale was tested among the parents of children aged 8 to 12 years with epilepsy and asthma, and good internal consistency and test–retest reliability were found. The third instrument is a 20-item measure completed by children themselves which addresses their anxieties about having seizures. Both the CATIS and the Child Concerns About Seizures Scale are welcome additions to the quality-of-life arena, because they are completed by children themselves, rather than relying on information obtained from parents.

The Dutch Study Group of Epilepsy in Childhood[73] has recently published two scales, both of which are intended for completion by parents. The first is a 19-item seizure severity scale which is a modified version of the adult seizure severity scale developed by Baker *et al.* in Liverpool.[36] The second is a

20-item scale designed to measure anti-epileptic side-effects in children. Both scales show good evidence of psychometric soundness, although information about their responsiveness to change is currently unavailable.

Another recently developed measure is the Impact of Childhood Illness Scale of Hoare and Russell.[74] This is a 30-item measure of quality of life in chronic childhood epilepsy, and it covers four broad areas, namely the impact of treatment, the impact on the child's development and adjustment, the impact on the parents and the impact on the family. It is completed by the parents, who rate each item on two dimensions – frequency and importance. Pilot validation work has provided preliminary evidence to support the usefulness of the scale, and further research is now in progress to assess its applicability in a larger and more representative group of children with epilepsy.

A version of the WPSI known as the Adolescent Psychosocial Seizure Inventory (APSI) has been available since 1991.[75] The QOLIE Group has also recently developed an instrument for adolescents with epilepsy, called the QOLIE-AD.[76] Item selection was based on interviews and focus groups with adolescents with mild, moderate and severe epilepsy, in order to represent the wide spectrum of problems faced by these young people. Test data from 194 adolescents were augmented by a brief parent-completed questionnaire in order to assess the level of agreement between parents and their teenage offspring. The test questionnaires included the CATIS and a stigma scale developed for adolescents, as well as standard mastery and self-esteem scales. Significant differences were found for CATIS and mastery across seizure severity groups, but not for self-esteem. Further work is needed to evaluate the responsiveness of the QOLIE-AD to changes in status or treatment.

The future of quality-of-life research in epilepsy

As we have shown, there is an increasing number of quality-of-life measures for epilepsy, some of which are better validated than others. It may be that certain measures eventually come to be seen as 'gold standards'. Recently, an attempt to identify potentially useful measures was made by a group of epilepsy experts, who rated 11 generic and epilepsy-specific quality-of-life instruments on five different dimensions.[77] In line with current thinking, the raters concluded that scales which were 'essentially "subjective", driven by patients' needs and assessing items selected by patients, would seem to be preferred'. As further information becomes available, it will be important to review and revise this initial list, but the rationale for it will have considerable appeal for non-experts in the outcomes field. Some degree of consensus concerning which are the most useful quality-of-life measures for epilepsy will also allow for standardisation across studies, which may in turn facilitate between-trial comparisons of quality-of-life data and meta-analyses of different study results. In the field of epilepsy, as elsewhere, there is great enthusiasm but also some scepticism about the value of quality-of-life assessment. However, acceptance of the limitations of seizure frequency as the only measure of outcome ensures that interest in the measurement of quality of life is unlikely to diminish in the foreseeable future.

References

1 Scambler G (1993) Epilepsy and quality of life research. *J R Soc Med.* **86**: 449–50.

2 Meador KJ (1993) Research use of the new quality-of-life in epilepsy inventory. *Epilepsia.* **34 (Supplement 4)**: S34–8.

3 Hermann BP (1998) The evolution of health-related quality of life assessment in epilepsy. *Qual Life Res.* **4**: 87–100.

4 Hermann BP (1992) Quality of life in epilepsy. *J Epilepsy.* **5**: 153–65.

5 Chaplin JE, Yepez R, Shorvon S and Floyd M (1991) A quantitative approach to measuring the social effects of epilepsy. *Neuroepidemiology.* **9**: 151–8.

6 Chaplin JE, Yepez Lasso R, Shorvon SD and Floyd M (1992) National general practice study of epilepsy: the social and psychological effects of a recent diagnosis of epilepsy. *BMJ*. **304**: 1416–18.

7 Gilliam F, Kuzniecky R, Faught E, Black L, Carpenter G and Schrodt R (1997) Patient-validated content of epilepsy-specific quality of life measurement. *Epilepsia*. **38**: 233–6.

8 Hauser WA and Annegers JF (1993) Epidemiology of epilepsy. In: J Laidlaw, A Richens and D Chadwick (eds) *A Textbook of Epilepsy* (4e). Churchill Livingstone, Edinburgh.

9 Chadwick D (1994) Epilepsy. *J Neurol Neurosurg Psychiatry*. **57**: 264–77.

10 International League Against Epilepsy (1989) *International Classification of Epilepsies and Epilepsy Syndromes*. Raven Press, New York.

11 International League Against Epilepsy (1981) Proposal for revised clinical and electroencephalographic classification of epileptic seizures. *Epilepsia*. **22**: 489–501.

12 Porter RJ (1993) Classification of epileptic seizures and epileptic syndromes. In: J Laidlaw, A Richens and D Chadwick (eds) *A Textbook of Epilepsy* (4e). Churchill Livingstone, Edinburgh.

13 Hauser WA and Hesdorffer DC (1990) *Epilepsy: Frequency, Causes and Consequences*. Epilepsy Foundation of America, Landover, MD.

14 Medical Research Council Antiepileptic Drug Withdrawal Study Group (1991) A randomised study of antiepileptic drug withdrawal in patients with epilepsy in remission. *Lancet*. **337**: 1175–80.

15 Jacoby A, Johnson A and Chadwick DW (1992) Psychosocial outcomes of antiepileptic drug discontinuation. *Epilepsia*. **33**: 1123–31.

16 Temkin O (1971) *The Falling Sickness*. Johns Hopkins Press, Baltimore, MD.

17 Caveness WF and Gallup GH (1980) A survey of public attitudes towards epilepsy in 1979 with an indication of trends over the past thirty years. *Epilepsia.* **21**: 509–18.

18 Canger R and Cornaggia C (1985) Public attitudes towards epilepsy in Italy: results of a survey and comparison with USA and West German data. *Epilepsia.* **26**: 221–6.

19 Schneider JW and Conrad P (1981) Medical and sociological typologies: the case of epilepsy. *Soc Sci Med.* **15A**: 211–19.

20 Schneider JW and Conrad P (1983) *Having Epilepsy: The Experience and Control of Illness.* Temple University Press, Philadelphia, PA.

21 Scambler G and Hopkins A (1986) Being epileptic: coming to terms with stigma. *Sociol Health Illness.* **8**: 26–43.

22 Scambler G (1989) *Epilepsy.* Tavistock, London.

23 Jacoby A (1994) Felt versus enacted stigma: a concept revisited. *Soc Sci Med.* **38**: 261–74.

24 Baker GA, Brooks J, Buck D and Jacoby A (2000) Stigma of epilepsy: findings from a European study. *Epilepsia.* In press.

25 Dell JL (1986) Social dimensions of epilepsy: stigma and response. In: S Whitman and HB Hermann (eds) *Psychopathology in Epilepsy: Social Dimensions.* Oxford University Press, Oxford.

26 Vickrey BG, Hays RD, Graber J, Rausch R, Engel J and Brook RH (1992) A health-related quality-of-life instrument for patients evaluated for epilepsy surgery. *Med Care.* **30**: 299–319.

27 Devinsky O, Vickrey BG, Cramer J *et al.* (1995) Development of the Quality of Life in Epilepsy Inventory. *Epilepsia.* **36**: 1089–104.

28 Baker GA, Jacoby A, Smith D, Dewey M and Chadwick DW (1994) Quality of life in epilepsy: the Liverpool initiative. In: MR Trimble and WE Dodson (eds) *Epilepsy and Quality of Life.* Raven Press, New York.

29 Kendrick AM and Trimble MR (1994) Repertory grid in the assessment of quality of life in patients with epilepsy:

the quality-of-life assessment schedule. In: MR Trimble and WE Dodson (eds) *Epilepsy and Quality of Life*. Raven Press, New York.

30 Dodrill CB, Batzel LW, Queisser HR and Temkin N (1980) An objective method for the assessment of psychological and social problems among epileptics. *Epilepsia*. **21**: 123–35.

31 Dodrill CB and Batzel LW (1995) Abstract: the Washington Psychosocial Seizure Inventory: new developments in the light of the quality-of-life concept. *Epilepsia*. **36**: S220.

32 Ware JE and Sherbourne CD (1992) The MOS 36-item Short-Form Health Survey (SF-36). I. Conceptual framework and item selection. *Med Care*. **30**: 473–83.

33 O'Donaghue MF, Duncan JS and Sander JWAS (1998) The subjective handicap of epilepsy: a new approach to measuring treatment outcome. *Brain*. **121**: 317–43.

34 Smith DF, Baker GA, Davies G, Dewey M and Chadwick DW. Outcomes of add-on treatment with Lamotrigine in partial epilepsy. *Epilepsia*. **34**: 312–22.

35 Baker GA, Smith DF, Dewey M, Jacoby A and Chadwick DW (1993) The initial development of a health-related quality-of-life model as an outcome measure in epilepsy. *Epilepsy Res*. **16**: 65–81.

36 Baker GA, Smith DF, Dewey M, Morrow J, Crawford PM and Chadwick DW (1991) The development of a seizure severity scale as an outcome measure in epilepsy. *Epilepsy Res*. **8**: 245–51.

37 Jacoby A, Baker GA, Smith DF, Dewey M and Chadwick DW (1993) Measuring the impact of epilepsy: the development of a novel scale. *Epilepsy Res*. **16**: 83–8.

38 Baker GA, Jacoby A, Smith DF, Dewey ME and Chadwick DW (1994) Development of a novel scale to assess life fulfilment as part of the further refinement of a quality-of-life model for epilepsy. *Epilepsia*. **35**: 591–6.

39 Baker GA, Jacoby A, Francis P and Chadwick DW (1995) The Liverpool Adverse Drug Events Profile. *Epilepsia*. **36** (**Supplement 3**): S179.

40   Gilham R, Baker G and Thompson P (1996) Standardisation of a self-report questionnaire for use in evaluating cognitive, affective and behavioural side-effects of anti-epileptic drug treatments. *Epilepsy Res.* **24**: 47-55.

41   Brown SW and Thomlinson LL (1982) Anticonvulsant side-effects: a self-report questionnaire for use in community surveys. *Br J Gen Pract.* **18**: 147–51.

42   Abetz L, Jacoby A, Baker GA and McNulty P (2000) Patient-based assessments of quality of life in newly diagnosed epilepsy patients. *Epilepsia.* In press.

43   Baker GA, Jacoby A and Berney T (1994) Abstract: development of an instrument to assess quality of life in children with epilepsy and learning disability. *Epilepsia.* **35** (**Supplement 7**): 47.

44   Jacoby A, Baker G, Bryant-Comstock L, Phillips S and Bamford C (1996) Lamotrigine add-on therapy is associated with improvement in mood in patients with severe epilepsy. *Epilepsia.* **37** (**Supplement 5**): S202.

45   Selai CE and Trimble MR (1995) Quality of life based on repertory grid technique (abstract). *Epilepsia.* **36** (**Supplement 3**): S220.

46   Selai C and Trimble MR (1998) Quality of life before and after temporal lobectomy. *Epilepsia.* **39** (**Supplement 2**): S63.

47   Kendrick AM (1993) *Repertory Grid Technique in the Assessment of Quality of Life in Patients with Epilepsy.* PhD Thesis, University of London, London.

48   Hays RD (1995) Directions for future research. *Qual Life Res.* **4**: 179–80.

49   Langfitt JT (1995) Comparison of the psychometric characteristics of three quality-of-life measures in intractable epilepsy. *Qual Life Res.* **4**: 101–14.

50   Wiebe S, Rose K, Derry P and McMachlan R (1997) Outcome assessment in epilepsy: comparative responsiveness of quality of life and psychosocial instruments. *Epilepsia.* **38**: 430–38.

51 Bergner M, Bobbitt RA, Pollard WE, Martin DP and Gilson BS (1976) The Sickness Impact Profile: validation of a health status measure. *Med. Care.* **14**: 57–67.

52 Guyatt GH, Eagle DJ, Sackett B *et al.* (1993) Measuring quality of life in the frail elderly. *J Clin Epidemiol.* **46**: 1433–44.

53 Wagner AK, Keller SD, Kosinski M *et al.* (1995) Advances in methods for assessing the impact of epilepsy and anti-epileptic drug therapy on patients' health-related quality of life. *Qual Life Res.* **4**: 115–34.

54 Pearlin L and Schooler C (1978) The structure of coping. *J Health Soc Behav.* **19**: 2-21.

55 Vickrey BG, Hays RD and Spritzer KL (1993) Methodological issues in QOL assessment for epilepsy surgery. In: DW Chadwick, GA Baker and A Jacoby (eds) *Quality of Life and Quality of Care in Epilepsy. Update 1993.* Royal Society of Medicine, London.

56 Deyo RA, Diehr P and Patrick DL (1991) Reproducibility and responsiveness of health status measures: statistics and strategies for evaluation. *Control Clin Trials.* **12**: S142–58.

57 Hays RD, Vickrey BG, Hermann BP *et al.* (1995) Agreement between self-reports and proxy reports of quality of life in epilepsy patients. *Qual Life Res.* **4**: 159–68.

58 Jaeschke R, Singer J and Guyatt G (1989) Measurements of health status: ascertaining the minimally important difference. *Control Clin Trials.* **10**: 407–15.

59 Juniper EF, Guyatt GH, Willan A and Griffith LE (1994) Determining a minimal important change in a disease-specific quality-of-life questionnaire. *J Clin Epidemiol.* **47**: 81–7.

60 Wagner AK and Vickrey BG (1995) The routine use of health-related quality-of-life measures in the care of patients with epilepsy: rationale and research agenda. *Qual Life Res.* **4**: 169–77.

61 Rapp S, Shumaker S, Smith T, Gibson P and Berzon R (1998) Adaptation and evaluation of the Liverpool Seizure

Severity Scale and Liverpool QOL Battery for American epilepsy patients. *Qual Life Res.* **7**: 353–63.

62 Collings J (1990) Psychosocial well-being and epilepsy: an empirical study. *Epilepsia.* **31**: 418–26.

63 Jacoby A (1992) Epilepsy and the quality of everyday life. Findings from a study of people with well-controlled epilepsy. *Soc Sci Med.* **43**: 657–66.

64 Baker GA, Jacoby A, Buck D, Stalgis C and Monnet D (1997) Quality of life of people with epilepsy: a European study. *Epilepsia.* **38**: 353–62.

65 Buck D, Jacoby A and Baker GA (2000) Cross-cultural differences in quality of life in epilepsy: findings from a European study. *Qual Life Res.* In press.

66 Dodrill CB, Arnett JL and Hayes AG (1996) Gabapentin monotherapy: quality-of-life evaluation during a double-blind, multicenter study in patients with medically refractory partial seizures (abstract). *Epilepsia.* **37**: S10.

67 Cramer JA, Perrine K, Devinsky O and Meador K (1996) A brief questionnaire to screen for quality of life in epilepsy: the QOLIE-10. *Epilepsia.* **37**: 577–82.

68 Wagner AK, Ehrenberg BL, Tran TA, Bungay KM, Cynn DJ and Rogers WH (1997) Patient-based health status measurement in clinical practice: a study of its impact on epilepsy patients' care. *Qual Life Res.* **6**: 329–41.

69 Austin JK, Shelton Smith M, Risinger MW and McNelis AM (1994) Childhood epilepsy and asthma: comparison of quality of life. *Epilepsia.* **35**: 608–15.

70 Austin JK, Huster GA, Dunn DW and Risinger MW (1996) Adolescents with active or inactive epilepsy or asthma: a comparison of quality of life. *Epilepsia.* **37**: 1228–37.

71 Austin JK and Huberty TJ (1993) Development of the Child Attitude Towards Illness Scale. *J Pediatr Psychol.* **18**: 467–80.

72 Austin JK, Patterson JM and Huberty TJ (1991) Development of the Coping Health Inventory for Children. *J Pediatr Nurs.* **6**: 166–74.

73 Carpay HA, Arts WFM, Vermeulen J *et al.* (1996) Parent-completed scales for measuring seizure severity and severity of side-effects of anti-epileptic drugs in childhood epilepsy: development and psychometric analysis. *Epilepsy Res.* **24**: 173–81.

74 Hoare P and Russell M (1995) The quality of life of children with chronic epilepsy and their families: preliminary findings with a new assessment measure. *Dev Med Child Neurol.* **37**: 689–96.

75 Batzel LW, Dodrill CB, Dubinskey BL *et al.* (1991) An objective method for the assessment of psychosocial problems in adolescents with epilepsy. *Epilepsia.* **32**: 202–11.

76 Cramer JA, Westbrook L and Devinsky O (2000) Evaluation of an instrument to assess quality of life in epilepsy for adolescents (QOLIE-AD). *Epilepsia.* In press.

77 Dodson WE and Trimble MR (1994) Epilogue: quality of life in epilepsy. In: MR Trimble and WE Dodson (eds) *Epilepsy and Quality of Life.* Raven Press, New York.

78 Cramer JA (1994) Quality of life for people with epilepsy. *Neurol Clin.* **12**: 1–13.

79 Hunt S, McKenna SP, McEwan J, Williams J and Papp E (1981) The Nottingham Health Profile: subjective health status and medical consultations. *Soc Sci Med.* **15**A: 221–9.

80 Zigmond AS and Snaith RP (1983) The Hospital Anxiety and Depression Scale. *Acta Psychiatr Scand.* **67**: 361–70.

81 Bradburn NM (1969) *The Structure of Psychological Well-Being.* Aldine Press, Chicago.

82 Rosenberg M (1965) *Society and the Adolescent Self-Image.* Princeton University Press, Princeton, NJ.

7
Alzheimer's disease

Khaled Amar

Introduction and epidemiology of Alzheimer's disease

It now almost a century since Alzheimer's first description of the clinical and pathological features of the disease that now bears his name. Alzheimer's disease was originally thought to be a rare cause of presenile dementia, but is now widely regarded as the most common cause of dementia, responsible for at least 50% of all cases.

Studies examining the incidence and prevalence of Alzheimer's disease are influenced by methodological issues such as the diagnostic criteria employed and the type of population examined (e.g. community-based or institution-based samples). A meta-analysis of published European studies examining the frequency and distribution of Alzheimer's disease reported no significant difference in the prevalence of this disease between various European studies.[1] The overall prevalence was reported to be 0.02% for ages 30–59 years, 0.3% for ages 60–69 years, 3.1% for ages 70–79 years and 10.8% for ages 80–89 years. In some populations the prevalence of Alzheimer's disease was reported to be consistently higher in older women. A more recent meta-analysis by Jorm and Jolly, which included studies from other continents, reported that the incidence of Alzheimer's disease increases linearly with age up to the age of 90 years.[2] However, East Asian countries were noted to have a lower incidence of Alzheimer's disease than Europe and the USA, although the exponential rise with age tended to be steeper.

Symptoms

The commonest presenting symptom in Alzheimer's disease is short-term memory loss. This leads to complaints from the patient, and more frequently from carers, of such problems as constantly losing personal possessions, forgetting appointments, and repeating oneself in conversation. Disorientation in time is also a common early problem, while disorientation in space – where the affected person gets lost in familiar surroundings, such as their own home – usually occurs in more advanced disease. Depression is common in early Alzheimer's disease and leads to symptoms such as loss of interest in pleasurable activities, early morning waking and weight loss. Language problems include expressive and later receptive dysphasia, resulting in increasing difficulty in communication. Apraxia frequently develops in moderate dementia, and results in difficulty in performing complex movements such as dressing, cooking or using 'gadgets' such as a TV remote control. Behavioural symptoms such as delusions and hallucinations occur in a certain proportion of patients with Alzheimer's disease, but agitation is more common, and is usually due to sheer frustration arising from poor memory and difficulties in communication. However, aggressive behaviour, particularly physical aggression, is rare. The development of agnosia results in inability to recognise familiar objects and faces. Personality changes such as disinhibited and inappropriate behaviour are rare, and when present early in the course of dementia would be suggestive of fronto-temporal dementia rather than Alzheimer's disease. In the advanced stages of Alzheimer's disease, the patient is almost completely mute and immobile, requiring total nursing care. Weight loss is common, and patients usually succumb to the sequelae of immobility and frailty, such as respiratory infections.

Treatment

There is currently no curative treatment for Alzheimer's disease. A cure for this disease will probably not become available until we have a better understanding of the exact pathogenesis of the disease. This would allow us to intervene at specific points of the pathogenic pathway in order to arrest the progression of the disease or, even better, to prevent it.

Depression is common in Alzheimer's disease, and is readily amenable to treatment. The use of the selective serotonin reuptake inhibitor (SSRI) antidepressants is preferable to the administration of tricyclic anticholinergics, as the latter can (at least theoretically) interfere with cholinergic transmission. Acetylcholine is an essential neurotransmitter for cognitive function and behaviour, and there is strong evidence of a significant deficit in cholinergic transmission in Alzheimer's disease.[3] This is the rationale for using drugs that promote cholinergic transmission in order to improve cognitive function. The anticholinesterase drug tacrine was the first drug to be licensed for the treatment of Alzheimer's disease, but its adverse effects, particularly liver toxicity and cholinergic symptoms, have limited its usefulness.[4] More recently, other anticholinesterases, such as donepezil (Aricept) and rivastigmine (Exelon), have been introduced and are generally better tolerated.[5,6]

Behaviour problems such as delusions, hallucinations and agitation can be very distressing to both patient and carer. However, before embarking on any drug treatment, a search for an organic cause or precipitating factors for these symptoms is essential. Symptoms such as agitation and aggression can simply be a manifestation of a medical problem such as urinary retention, constipation or pain. Tackling these problems will usually resolve the behavioural symptoms. Even if there is no clear medical explanation, the use of non-pharmacological approaches, such as reassurance and distraction, should always be tried before prescribing neuroleptic medication. If these drugs have to be used, the dosage should always be kept to a minimum and the treatment reviewed periodically so that it can be stopped at the earliest opportunity. Finally, it is important when we consider treatments not to forget the carers and how best to support them. They are often under tremendous stress as they try to come to terms with the impact of this devastating disease.

Clinical measurement

A number of scales are used to measure clinical features such as cognitive function, behavioural symptoms and activities of daily living. These scales are essential for quantifying the degree of impairment in these areas as a result of the disease, and for measuring the response to treatments or interventions. The ideal scale needs to fulfil the following criteria:

- validity – measuring what it claims to measure

- sensitivity – responsive to meaningful change

- reliability – reproducible on retesting and between different raters

- precision – having a wide range with no ceiling or floor effect

- feasibility – acceptable to the patient and practical (e.g. not too time-consuming or expensive to administer).

Cognitive assessment scales

Cognitive tests are the primary measure of efficacy in clinical trials evaluating new therapies for Alzheimer's disease. A substantial number of different cognitive neuropsychological assessment instruments are in use.

The Mini-Mental State Examination (MMSE) is a brief interviewer-administered test of global cognitive function, consisting of 30 questions, introduced initially as a screening tool for dementia by Folstein et al.[7] It is often used in drug trials as a secondary measure of cognitive function and for staging the severity of dementia. The MMSE is simple to administer, taking approximately 10 minutes to complete, but is relatively crude and insensitive.

The Alzheimer's Disease Assessment Scale contains a cognitive subscale (ADAS-cog) in the form of a battery of individual cognitive tests that are thought to be sensitive to changes in Alzheimer's disease.[8] The areas that are examined include memory, orientation in time and space, praxis and language skills. The result is expressed in an overall summary score. The ADAS-cog is an error score, ranging from 0 to 70, that takes approximately 1 hour to administer. This instrument has been widely used in recent trials, and has been shown to be valid, revealing significant differences between active drugs and placebo in a number of Alzheimer's disease drug trials. For example, Greenberg et al. found a significant difference in patients with Alzheimer's disease receiving donepezil compared to placebo over a 6-week period in cognitive function assessed by ADAS-cog.[9] Versions of the instrument also exist in languages other than English, such as French, Spanish and German, facilitating its use in multicentre trials.

The Severe Impairment Battery (SIB) was designed specifically for patients with moderate to severe dementia, in which patients have great difficulty in communicating and are unable to comply with conventional cognitive tests.[10] The tests rely on single words or simple one-step commands. The SIB covers several cognitive domains, and has been shown to be sensitive in moderate dementia.

Behavioural rating scales

There is a range of clinical scales intended to cover behavioural problems such as agitation, delusions, hallucinations and depression. It is important to quantify and grade these behavioural symptoms, as anti-dementia drugs may have an effect on behaviour as well as on cognitive function.

The Alzheimer's Disease Assessment Scale/non-cognitive subscale (ADAS-non-cog) is usually combined with the ADAS-cog scale to yield a total ADAS score. The rating is made by the person administering the test, and is dependent on behaviour during the test. It covers the areas of depression, tearfulness, concentration, delusions, hallucinations, tremors, pacing, motor activity, appetite and unco-operativeness.[8] The score is in the form of a 6-point severity scale ranging from 0 to 5.

The Behaviour Rating Scale for Dementia of the Consortium to Establish a Registry for Alzheimer's Disease (CERAD BRSD) is in the form of a standardised semi-structured interview administered to caregivers.[11] It is intended to assess behavioural abnormalities and it emphasises psychopathology. It covers depressive features, psychotic features, defective self-regulation, irritability/agitation, vegetative features, apathy, aggression and affective lability. The questionnaire is available in a 46-item version or a shorter 17-item version, and has been shown to have good reliability.

The Short Observation Method (SOM) records the times spent by the individual on specific activities.[12] The method involves recording the activities of the patient every 10 seconds, through observation over a period of time, using different codes. Social contacts and responses are also recorded. Although attention has been given to validity and reliability, there seems to be little evidence available on sensitivity to change. The time and resources required to use such methods are very substantial, so there may be real limitations on the feasibility of such an approach in, for example, large multicentre trials.

The Behaviour Pathology in Alzheimer's Disease (BEHAVE-AD) Scale assesses behaviour in seven domains, namely paranoid and delusional ideation, hallucinations, activity disturbances, aggressiveness, diurnal rhythm disturbances, affective disturbances, anxieties and phobias.[13] Abnormal behaviour is rated as mild, moderate or severe. More recent evidence from factor analysis of data from a consecutive series of patients with Alzheimer's disease suggests that the instrument addresses five underlying aspects of psychopathology, namely agitation and anxiety, psychosis, aggression, depression and activity disturbance.[14]

Activities of daily living scales

Measurement of the degree of dependency in patients with Alzheimer's disease is important for determining the effectiveness of treatments or interventions, and also for judging how much support a patient needs, and in which areas.

The Progressive Deterioration Scale (PDS) has been described as a quality-of-life measure, so it will be considered in more detail in a later section of the chapter.[15] However, it may also be regarded as a measure of activities of daily living. It covers areas such as ability to travel alone, confusion in familiar settings, participation in leisure activities and household chores, self-care and social functioning. It has been well validated in Alzheimer's disease, and was shown to have good reliability and sensitivity. As described below, it is now among the more commonly used measures in clinical trials.

The Physical Self-Maintenance Scale (PSMS) assesses basic activities including feeding, dressing, toileting, grooming, bathing and ambulation.[16] Scoring is on a 5-point rating scale, and observations can be made by different members of the healthcare team, either in the community or in institutions. There is only limited evidence of the sensitivity and reliability of the PSMS.

The Instrumental Activities of Daily Living (IADL) was also designed by Lawton and colleagues.[16] It examines more complex activities that require a higher level of independent functioning. It assesses performance in the activities of shopping, telephoning, food preparation, housekeeping, laundry, transportation, finances and responsibility for medication. It is scored by the caregiver (with a score range of 4–30). There is only limited evidence of the sensitivity and reliability of the IADL.

Health status measurement

Health status measurement refers to the measurement of quality of life. The pharmaceutical industry, including manufacturers of anti-dementia drugs, is now required to provide evidence that its treatments are of real and meaningful benefit to patients and can improve the quality of their lives. Outcome measures for the assessment of quality of life in Alzheimer's disease are now widely regarded as being essential for evaluating and monitoring a patient's status, for selecting and monitoring the patient's response to certain treatments or interventions, and for gaining a better understanding of the disease itself.

Quality of life is a multifaceted concept that is both objective and, more importantly, subjective. It is influenced by biological, socio-economic, psychological and environmental factors. Health and public-health researchers have concentrated on health-related quality of life, but the latter cannot be considered in isolation from all the other factors. Quality-of-life assessment has become widely accepted in the field of pharmaco-economics, which assesses the overall costs and benefits of different interventions, such as drugs. Certain forms of quality-of-life measure are also intended to facilitate comparisons of effectiveness across different diseases.

An ideal quality-of-life scale needs to be valid, reliable, responsive and practical. Devising such a scale is particularly difficult in the case of Alzheimer's disease, both due to impaired cognitive function and the resulting difficulty in communication, and because of the impact of disease processes on the patient's judgement, which may be particularly impaired in patients with more advanced dementia. This means that, with advancing cognitive impairment, such measurement inevitably relies increasingly on a proxy informant rather than the patient. This is not an ideal situation, as the patient's perspective of a good quality of life may be different to that of the informant. Important areas of future research need to ask how much insight a patient with moderate or severe Alzheimer's disease has, and whether insight is dependent on cognitive function.

Generic measures of quality of life

A number of generic measures have been examined for their applicability in the context of Alzheimer's disease. One of the most commonly used instruments in other contexts is the Sickness Impact Profile (SIP), which consists of 136 items which can be either interviewer administered to the patient or carer, or self-administered.[17] It provides scores of 12 subscales that may also be combined into two overall dimensions – a physical dimension (body care and movement, mobility and ambulation) and a psychosocial dimension (emotional behaviour, social interaction, alertness and communication) – with a third independent group of subscales (sleep and rest, home management, work, recreation and pastimes, and eating).

The SIP has been validated in mild Alzheimer's disease, and was shown to be reliable. A number of modified forms of this instrument have appeared. The UK SIP (UK-SIP) was adapted using British English for use in the UK. The Summary UK-SIP was reduced to only 14 items, and is self-administered, with response categories in the form of visual analogue scales. The

SIP for Nursing Homes (SIP-NH) was modified to evaluate nursing home patients, with the number of items reduced from 136 to only 66. However, shortened versions of the instrument have received little use.

The SIP has been used in a clinical trial of levocarnitine for dementia.[18] It was administered to the patient's regular carer who acted as a proxy respondent. No evidence of the impact of the drug on SIP scores was observed and, as is often the case in such studies, it is difficult to determine whether such results are due to ineffectiveness of the intervention rather than to insensitivity of the measure.

The most widely used generic instrument is the 36 Short-Form Health Survey Questionnaire (SF-36), which consists of 36 items that provide an assessment of general health.[19] Its scales may be grouped to provide overall scores in two main domains − physical health (formed from scales of physical functioning, physical role, bodily pain and general health) and mental health (formed from scales of vitality, social functioning, emotional role and mental health) − as well as self-evaluation of health over the past year. The SF-36 is a self-completed questionnaire. The items of the scales are summed to produce scale scores ranging from 0 (worst possible health) to 100 (best possible health). It has been well validated, but there are still concerns about whether the instrument is appropriate in content and acceptable in format to older people.[20] Moreover, there appear to be potential problems with regard to comprehension among older individuals with any cognitive impairment.[21]

Pearlman and Uhlmann developed an instrument to elicit global self-assessments of quality of life on a 6-point scale specifically for use with older people with chronic illnesses.[22] This approach has been adapted by Mezey et al. for completion by spouses to rate the quality of life of individuals with dementia.[23] The areas covered include memory, mood, physical health, functional ability, interpersonal relationships, psychological well-being, life satisfaction, participation in religious activities, environmental comfort and physical discomfort. Walker *et al.* point out that there are potential methodological problems in adapting an instrument developed for self-completion by patients to a format where it is intended to be used by a proxy respondent (such as a carer), and the instrument requires further validation in this novel mode of administration.[24]

Kaplan *et al.* developed an instrument originally known as the Index of Well-Being (IWB), but more recently named the Quality of Well-Being (QWB) Scale.[25] It is an interview-based instrument which, by a combination of screening followed by more specific questions, obtains information about symptoms and function, with functional assessment of three specific domains, namely mobility, physical activity and social activity. Individuals are assigned an overall health status as a result of information about symptoms and function, and these health states are associated with weighted values obtained from separate measurement of panels' preferences regarding different health states. The QWB has been used to compare different forms of residential and care arrangements for individuals with dementia.[26] However, it is of importance that the data for this study were collected by means of another instrument and an algorithm was used to convert the results into QWB scores. This is a somewhat cumbersome and indirect way of using an instrument.

More recently, it has been argued that conventional questionnaires impose predetermined issues on respondents because of their standardised format of questions. In response to such criticisms, the Schedule for the Evaluation of Individual Quality of Life (SEIQOL) was developed.[27] It is administered as a semi-structured interview in which subjects are asked to nominate without prompting five areas of daily living which they consider to be important determinants of their quality of life. Scoring is by the subjects themselves using visual analogue scales. Coen *et al.* administered the SEIQOL to individuals with dementia and found that many respondents have problems of comprehension that result in inaccurate completion of the interview.[28] The more severe the patients' cognitive impairment, the greater the degree of difficulty experienced. Walker *et al.* have argued that the SEIQOL may therefore require too high a level of insight on the part of respondents to be at all feasible for any other but the most mildly impaired patients with dementia.[24]

Disease-specific measures of quality of life

As in most other fields of medicine, it has proved necessary to develop instruments intended to be used specifically for patients with dementia and Alzheimer's disease, in order that the content of instruments may be of maximal relevance to patients with Alzheimer's disease.

Thus the Progressive Deterioration Scale (PDS) was specifically designed for use in patients with Alzheimer's disease and emerged initially, as described above, as a measure of activities of daily living.[15] It consists of 27 items in the form of visual analogue scales, and is intended to be completed by the carer of a patient with dementia. It has been shown to discriminate between older respondents with and without dementia.[23] The PDS has been successfully used as a measure of quality of life in drug trials of the anticholinesterase drugs tacrine and rivastigmine, with results showing, for example, significant differences between active drug and placebo.[4,29]

The Quality of Life-AD (QOL-AD) consists of 13 items to be completed by both the patient and their carer.[30] It covers the areas of physical condition, mood, concern about finances, relationships with friends and family, and an overall assessment of quality of life. It is unusual in the sense that, if possible, both the carer and the patient are required to complete equivalent versions, except that the patient's answers are obtained from interview and the carer's are obtained via a questionnaire. Total scores for the individual patient are obtained by adding the patient's and carer's scores, with the patient's score being given greater numerical weighting. A good correlation between patients' and carers' responses has been observed, and at least for patients with low to moderate levels of cognitive impairment, the reliability and validity of the instrument are very satisfactory. Given that the time required to complete the instrument is 5–10 minutes for carers and 10–15 minutes for patients, the instrument may be considered promising in terms of practical feasibility. It may therefore be potentially useful in Alzheimer's disease patients with mild and moderate dementia.

Brod et al. have produced another very promising instrument designed for use in a direct interview with patients with dementia.[31] They selected their potential questionnaire items from an initial series of focus groups with caregivers, professional healthcare providers and patients with dementia. An initial set of 96 candidate questionnaire items was reduced by standard psychometric techniques to a final version of the questionnaire with 29 items forming 5 scales, namely self-esteem, positive affect, negative affect, feelings of belonging and sense of aesthetics. The authors found that the resulting instrument showed the same reproducibility over a period of two weeks in groups of patients with both mild and moderate levels of cognitive impairment from dementia. The Dementia Quality of Life Instrument (DQOL) that emerged from the careful process of development and testing is unusual in that it identifies dimensions of quality of life that are of concern to patients with dementia that have not been emphasised in other work. For example, the aesthetics scale addresses pleasure derived from sensory awareness and appreciation of beauty in nature, music and the environment. As the authors comment, not only does this scale address a potentially positive dimension of well-being, but also suggests potentially beneficial social interventions to improve quality of life. Overall, Brod et al. recognise the extent of the problems involved in obtaining quality-of-life data from the cognitively impaired, and they suggest a mixed strategy in which more 'objective' dimensions such as daily activities, physical function and social interaction are best obtained via proxy report from other available instruments, whilst the DQOL provides unique evidence of 'subjective' domains such as sense of well-being and aesthetics.

For patients who are more severely cognitively impaired, inevitably attention continues to focus on improved observer-based scales. The Cognitively Impaired Life Quality (CILQ) Scale was devised to measure the quality of life of severely demented patients.[32] Nursing caregivers were asked to grade patients' quality of life on 29 items, each using a 5-point scale ranging from very good to very poor. The areas examined included social interaction, physical care, appearance of the patient to others, nutrition and pain. Further item-reduction analyses have resulted in a 14-item version that still addresses the same dimensions of quality of life as the fuller version, but is considered more feasible for routine clinical use. To date, evidence of validity comes from the finding that CILQ scale scores differed significantly in the predicted direction between patients with dementia in long-term care who were separately rated as having higher and lower levels of functioning.

Although it is not a primary focus of this chapter, the well-being of those who care for patients with dementia is a distinct and important issue. It is increasingly recognised that carers may experience substantial physical, emotional and social problems as a result of their role. Because of the mutual effects on well-being of the patient with dementia and their carer, it is essential for evaluations of the cost-effectiveness of interventions to broaden the scope of outcomes to include carers' well-being. One instrument that has been explicitly developed with this broader scope in mind is the Community Dementia Quality-of-Life Profile (CDQLP).[33] One part of this instrument focuses on the well-being of the patient with dementia, as assessed by the carer, while the second part focuses on the carer's own well-being. It consists of 33 items covering the areas of thinking and behaviour, family and social life, physical activities and other aspects of daily living. Evidence of the internal consistency and reproducibility of this instrument is encouraging, but evidence of its validity and sensitivity to change still needs to be demonstrated.

Conclusion

Alzheimer's disease is the commonest cause of dementia. It has a devastating effect on the quality of life of both the sufferers and their carers. The availability of good clinical and quality-of-life measures is essential in the search for effective treatments, and also for comparing different interventions. An effective treatment for Alzheimer's disease is meaningless if a significant improvement in the quality of life of patients and their carers cannot be demonstrated.

There are unique challenges in assessing constructs such as quality of life of individuals with significant cognitive impairment. It will always be necessary to involve observers such as the carer in this context. Nevertheless, it is striking how increasingly optimistic investigators have become about the scope for increasing the role of all but the most severely cognitively impaired patients in directly judging their own quality of life.

Although a large number of quality-of-life scales already exist, we are still searching for a scale that can be regarded as the gold standard in this area. The quality-of-life scales currently available still fall short of achieving all of the desired qualities, which must include validity, reliability, sensitivity to change, precision and feasibility. Some of the existing quality-of-life scales, such as the Sickness Impact Profile, the Progressive Deterioration Scale and the Quality of Life-AD, are very promising but need further testing in clinical trials for patients with dementia. In future, it may be a more fruitful strategy to try to modify and refine existing scales, rather than to design new ones. As Salek *et al.* have argued, further progress in this area will require both the application of basic psychometric techniques to ensure that instruments are identified with optimal measurement properties, and conceptual research to establish the key concerns of patients and their carers in relation to dementia.[34] The development of a growing number of drugs with potentially beneficial therapeutic effects has made the task of refining outcomes methodology in this area an imperative.

References

1 Rocca WA, Hofman A, Brayne C *et al.* (1991) Frequency and distribution of Alzheimer's disease in Europe: a collaborative study of 1980–1990 findings. *Ann Neurol.* **30**: 381–90.

2 Jorm A and Jolly D (1998) The incidence of dementia – a meta-analysis. *Neurology.* **51**: 728–33.

3 Wilcock GKW and Esiri MM (1982) Plaques, tangles and dementia – a quantitative study. *J Neurol Sci.* **56**: 343–56.

4 Knapp MJ, Knopman DS and Solomon PR (1994) A 30-week randomised controlled trial of high-dose tacrine in patients with Alzheimer's disease. *JAMA.* **271**: 985–91.

5 Rogers SL, Farlow MR, Doody RS, Mohs R and Friedhoff LT (1998) A 24-week, double-blind, placebo-controlled trial of donepezil in patients with Alzheimer's disease. Donepezil Study Group. *Neurology.* **50**: 136–45.

6 Corey-Bloom J, Annad R and Veach J (1998) A randomized trial evaluating the efficacy and safety of ENA 713 (rivastigmine tartrate), a new acetylcholinesterase inhibitor, in patients with mild to moderately severe Alzheimer's disease. *Int J Geriatr Psychopharmacol.* **1**: 55–65.

7 Folstein FM, Folstein SE and McHugh PR (1975) Mini-Mental State – a practical method for grading the cognitive state of patients for the clinician. *J Psychiatr Res.* **12**: 189–98.

8 Rosen WG, Mohs RC and Davis KL (1984) A new rating scale for Alzheimer's disease. *Am J Psychiatry.* **141**: 1356–64.

9 Greenberg S, Tennis M, Brown L *et al.* (2000) Donepezil therapy in clinical practice: a randomized crossover study. *Arch Neurology.* **57**: 94–9.

10 Saxton J, McGongle-Gibson KL and Swihart AA (1990) Assessment of the severely impaired patient: description and validation of a new neuropsychological test battery. *Psychol Assess.* **2**: 298–303.

11 Tariot PN, Mack JL, Patterson MB *et al.* (1995) The Behaviour Rating Scale for Dementia of the Consortium to Establish a Registry for Alzheimer's Disease. The Behavioral Pathology Committee of the Consortium to Establish a Registry for Alzheimer's Disease. *Am J Psychiatry.* **152**: 1349–57.

12 MacDonald A, Craig T and Warner L (1985) The development of a short observation method for the study of activity and contacts of old people in residential settings. *Psychol Med.* **15**: 167–72.

13 Reisberg B, Ferris SH and de Leon MJ (1982) The Global Deterioration Scale for assessment of primary degenerative dementia. *Am J Psychiatry.* **139**: 1136–9.

14 Harwood DG, Ownby RL, Barker WW and Duara R (1998) The behavioral pathology in Alzheimer's Disease Scale (BEHAVE-AD): factor structure among community-dwelling Alzheimer's disease patients. *Int J Geriatr Psychiatry.* **13**: 793–800.

15 DeJong R, Osterlund OW and Roy GW (1989) Measurement of quality-of-life changes in patients with Alzheimer's disease. *Clin Ther.* **11**: 545–54.

16 Lawton MP and Brody EM (1969) Assessment of older people: self-maintaining and instrumental activities of daily living. *Gerontologist.* **9**: 176–86.

17 Bergner M, Bobbitt RA, Kressel S, Pollard W, Gilson B and Morris J (1976) The Sickness Impact Profile: conceptual formulation and methodology for the development of health status measure. *Int J Health Serv.* **6**: 393–415.

18 Sano M, Bell K, Cote L *et al.* (1992) Double-blind parallel-design pilot study of acetyl levocarnitine in patients with Alzheimer's disease. *Arch Neurol.* **49**: 1137–41.

19 Brazier JE, Harper R, Jones NMB *et al.* (1992) Validating the SF-36 health survey questionnaire: new outcome measure for primary care. *BMJ.* **305**: 160–64.

20 Hill S, Harries U and Popay J (1996) Is the Short-Form 36 (SF-36) suitable for routine health outcomes assessment in

health care for older people? Evidence from preliminary work in community-based health services in England. *J Epidemiol Commun Health.* **50**: 94–8.

21 Parker S, Peet S, Jagger C, Farhan M and Castleden C (1998) Measuring health status in older patients: the SF-36 in practice. *Age Ageing.* **27**: 13–18.

22 Pearlman R and Uhlmann R (1988) Patient and physician perceptions of patient quality of life in chronic diseases. *J Gerontol.* **43**: M25–30.

23 Mezey M, Kluger M and Maislin G (1996) Life-sustaining treatment decisions by spouses of patients with Alzheimer's disease. *J Am Geriatr Soc.* **44**: 144–50.

24 Walker M, Salek S and Bayer A (1998) A review of quality of life in Alzheimer's disease. Part 1. Issues in assessing disease impact. *Pharmaco-economics.* **14**: 499–530.

25 Kaplan RM and Bush JW (1982) Health-related quality-of-life measurement for evaluation research and policy analysis. *Health Psychol.* **1**: 61–80.

26 Wimo A, Mattson B, Krakau I, Eriksson T, Nelvig A and Karlsson G (1995) Cost-utility analysis of group living in dementia care. *Int J Technol Assess Health Care.* **11**: 49–65.

27 O'Boyle C, McGee H, Hickey A, O'Malley K and Joyce C (1992) Individual quality of life in patients undergoing hip replacement. *Lancet.* **339**: 1088–91.

28 Coen R, O'Mahony D, O'Boyle C *et al.* (1993) Measuring the quality of life of dementia patients using the Schedule for the Evaluation of Individualised Quality of Life. *Ir J Psychol.* **14**: 154–63.

29 Vincent SA and Harvey RJ (1998) *The ADENA Programme. Clinical Advances in Drug Development: Alzheimer's Disease Trial Design.* Medpress, Sevenoaks.

30 Logsdon RG (1996) Quality of life in Alzheimer's disease: implications for research (abstract). *Gerontologist.* **36** (**Special Issue 1**): 278.

31 Brod M, Stewart A, Sands L and Walton P (1999) Conceptualization and measurement of quality of life in

dementia: the Dementia Quality of Life Rating Instrument (D-QOL). *Gerontologist.* **39**: 25–35.

32 DeLetter MC, Tully CL and Wilson JF (1995) Nursing staff perceptions of quality of life of cognitively impaired elders: instrumental development. *J Appl Gerontol.* **14**: 426–43.

33 Salek MS, Schwartzberg E and Bayer AJ (1996) Evaluating health-related quality of life in patients with dementia: development of a proxy self-administered questionnaire (abstract). *Pharm World Sci.* **18** (**5 Supplement A**): 6.

34 Salek MS, Walker M and Bayer A (1998) A review of quality of life in Alzheimer's disease. Part 2. Issues in assessing drug effects. *Pharmaco-economics.* **14**: 613–27.

8

Amyotrophic lateral sclerosis/motor neurone disease

Crispin Jenkinson, Ray Fitzpatrick and Michael Swash

Introduction

Amyotrophic lateral sclerosis (ALS) is a progressive fatal disorder with an incidence of about 2 in 100 000 per year, and a prevalence of about 6 in 100 000.[1] It is characterised by increasing weakness of the limb, trunk, ventilatory and bulbar muscles, usually without impairment of the sphincters, or of intellectual faculties. As a result, there is increasing dependency on the patient's family and other carers.[2] In the longer term, this will lead to a state of physical dependency and immobility. Despite the substantial impact of ALS/motor neurone disease (MND) upon patients, it is only very recently that work has been undertaken to assess systematically the impact in terms of subjective health status and quality of life. This chapter will outline the use of generic health status measures in the assessment of amyotrophic lateral sclerosis/motor neurone disease,[3] and will outline the development and validation of the first measure designed specifically for patients diagnosed with these conditions.

Clinimetric scales used in amyotrophic lateral sclerosis

The commonest primary outcome points in trials of treatment regimes for ALS/MND are muscle strength, pulmonary function and mortality. Perhaps the most widely known measure is the Norris ALS Scale,[4] which was designed to track clinical changes in ALS patients after treatment. This scale measures both impairments and disabilities. It provides scores for bulbar, respiratory, arm, trunk and leg domains, as well as a general domain that measures (among other things) fatigue and emotional health. The measure assigns weights of equal value to different aspects of patients' functioning, which does not seem appropriate in view of the fact that it also assesses areas of health state, such as bladder and bowel function, that are seldom influenced by ALS.[5] The Appel Scale is another widely used measure, and consists of assessments of bulbar involvement (speech and swallowing), respiratory involvement, muscle strength in the arms and legs, lower extremity function and upper extremity function. Assessments are made by clinical evaluation. The disparate scores obtained from the assessment are used to obtain a single total scale score. Although the construct validity of the measure has been supported by evidence of increasing scores on the overall index as the disease progresses,[6] such addition of the various assessments has been criticised as having limited meaning.[7] The most recent attempt to develop a clinimetric scale which is simple to use and can provide meaningful data is the ALS Functional Rating Scale (ALSFRS).[7] The ALSFRS is a 10-item functional inventory which was devised for use in therapeutic trials in ALS and covers the areas of speech, salivation, swallowing, handwriting, cutting food, dressing and hygiene, turning in bed, walking, climbing stairs and breathing. Each item is rated on a scale of 0 to 4 by the patient and/or their caregiver, yielding a maximum score of 40 points. The ALSFRS assesses patient levels of self-sufficiency in the areas of feeding, grooming, ambulation and communication. The ALSFRS has been validated both cross-sectionally and longitudinally against muscle strength testing, the Schwab and England Activities of Daily Living rating scale, the Clinical Global Impression of Change (CGIC) scale, and independent assessments of patient functional status. Evidence has also been provided for the ALS test–retest reliability and consistency of the ALSFRS in a large, multicentre clinical trial.[8] One weakness of the ALSFRS is that it grants disproportionate weighting to limb and bulbar, as compared to respiratory, dysfunction. A revised version of the ALSFRS, which incorporates additional assessments of dyspnoea, orthopnoea and the need for ventilatory support, has recently been introduced. The Revised ALSFRS (ALSFRS-R) retains the properties of the original scale and shows strong internal consistency and construct validity.[9] However, despite the excellent properties of the ALSFRS, the impact of newly developed therapies increasingly requires a broader assessment of outcome in terms of subjective health status. For example, the ASFRS does not attempt to assess the impact of ill health on emotional functioning or social functioning. Thus there is a need for measures of health status that provide a more subjective, and hence more complete, picture of the impact of the disease on patient functioning and well-being.

Generic measures of health status

The 36-item Short-Form Health Survey (SF-36) questionnaire[10] is perhaps the most widely used measure of general health status at present, and it has recently been evaluated for use in ALS/MND patients. In one study the progression of disability and the patients' perception of their health were assessed in a small group of MND patients ($n = 14$) for 6 months from the point of diagnosis or very soon afterwards, and compared with a group of patients of similar age with Parkinson's disease (PD). MND patients showed a far more rapid deterioration in health status on a number of clinical measures. At recruitment, perception of physical health was worse for both groups than for age- and sex-matched population norms. In both groups the SF-36 could not be used to monitor changes in perception of health because of floor effects on a number of domains.[11] However, these results conflict with those obtained from an American study which compared the results from the SF-36 with those obtained from the Tufts Quantitative Neuromuscular Exam (TQNE). This study examined the reliability and responsiveness of each measure, and compared the health status of individuals with ALS with that of the general population. Subjects ($n = 31$) completed the SF-36 and the TQNE at two time points within a period of 1 week in order to determine reliability. In addition, 17 subjects also completed both the TQNE and the SF-36 each month for 1 year after diagnosis of ALS in order to establish the relationship between the two assessment tools. This paper argued that both the TQNE and the SF-36 were reliable and responsive and appear to be important in the characterisation of patient status after ALS is diagnosed.[12]

The SF-36 is currently being used in the European ALS-Health Profile Study.[13] This is a large-scale study that is being undertaken throughout Europe to evaluate the health status of patients with ALS/MND. The evidence available to date suggests that there are floor effects, particularly in the 'physical role' dimension of the instrument. However, the SF-36 has recently been altered to overcome this problem, and the subsequent SF-36 version 2 may be a more appropriate instrument for evaluation of the consequences of ALS/MND.[14] A subset of items from the SF-36 has been used to construct the 12-item Health Survey Questionnaire (SF-12).[15] This questionnaire is being used in a large-scale survey in the USA (the ALS CARE programme). At present there is limited information on the appropriateness of this measure in this population, although the evidence to date suggests that it provides a similar picture of health status to the SF-36.[16]

Recent trials of ALS therapies have included the Sickness Impact Profile (SIP) to evaluate health-related quality of life, and the feasibility, psychometric properties and interpretation of the SIP have been evaluated in this setting. The SIP is a questionnaire containing 136 items, and it can provide an overall scale score and/or scores for 12 sub-dimensions as well as physical and psychosocial summary scores. In one study, the SIP was administered at baseline, 3, 6 and 9 months during a double-blind, placebo-controlled study of recombinant human insulin-like growth factor I. The frequency of missing SIP data and the administration time were recorded. Patients' scores on the Appel ALS Rating Scale were used to identify a stable subgroup for reliability testing and clinically distinct groups for validity testing. Internal consistency reliability and reproducibility were evaluated using Cronbach's alpha and intraclass correlation coefficients, respectively. Analysis-of-variance (ANOVA) models and t-tests were used to assess validity. Effect sizes and the responsiveness index were used to assess responsiveness. At baseline, 259 patients (97%) completed a 30-minute interview which included the SIP. At subsequent assessments, the response rates ranged from 92% to 97% and the mean administration time ranged from 25 to 27 minutes. The overall SIP score demonstrated high internal reliability and stability coefficients. Baseline overall SIP scores discriminated between patients in the two Appel ALS score-defined groups. Similarly, the mean overall change in SIP scores discriminated between patients progressing at different rates. With few exceptions, the dimension scores fulfilled similar criteria. Responsiveness statistics for the physical and overall SIP scores were lower at 3 months and higher at 6 and 9 months, as the disease progressed. The authors concluded that these findings support the validity of the SIP for assessing outcomes of ALS and its treatment in future clinical trials.[17] However, they claim that the study design which they adopted had limitations in assessing the usefulness of the SIP as a measure of psychosocial well-being, as the primary end-points of the trial were measures of physical function. Indeed, this limitation is present in other assessments of the SIP in ALS. For example, the Tufts Quantitative Neuromuscular Exam (TQNE) is a standardised tool for measuring muscle strength and pulmonary function in patients with ALS, and in a study of 524 ALS patients a significant relationship was found between TQNE and SIP scores, both cross-sectionally and over time.[18] Once again, this provides evidence for the ability of the SIP to measure physical functioning in ALS, but only limited evidence for its suitability for assessing psychosocial aspects of health state. None the less, the evidence available seems to suggest that the SIP is an appropriate tool for this patient group.

One obvious criticism of the SIP is that it takes considerable time to complete, and this can be demanding for patients with serious conditions such as ALS/MND. Consequently, a shorter version has been developed specifically for use with ALS/MND patients.[19] The authors examined SIP subscales and clinically derived item sets in relation to the TQNE CM in an attempt to define a briefer measure of quality of life for use in clinical trials. Two 'Mini-SIP' indices performed as well as the overall SIP in reflecting the impact of muscle weakness on ALS patients' quality of life. These were a combination of two SIP subscales (SIP-33) and a 19-item set of questions independently chosen by a panel of ALS specialists (SIP/ALS-19), respectively. The developers suggest that either index could potentially be useful in ALS clinical trials, but further evaluation of the measures is required. The SIP/ALS-19 is currently being used in a national ALS database (the ALS CARE programme), providing an opportunity to evaluate its utility prospectively against other quality-of-life measures in ALS patients.[16] To date, only limited data have become available on this shortened, disease-specific version of the SIP. Ideally, however, disease-specific measures are not adapted from existing measures but are designed 'from the ground up', and at present only one such measure exists – the 40-item ALS Assessment Questionnaire (ALSAQ-40). The development and validation of this new measure are outlined below.

The ALSAQ-40 disease-specific health status measure

In order to develop a disease-specific health status measure for ALS/MND, a three-stage development process was followed. In the first stage, in-depth semi-structured interviews with 18 patients presenting with ALS were tape-recorded. The sample size for this stage of the study was determined by the point at which no new significant themes appeared to emerge from the interviews. Patients presented with ALS across the breadth of the disease process, and at different ages. They were asked to describe the areas of their lives that had been influenced by ALS/MND. A list of aspects of life that were adversely affected by the disease was extracted from the transcribed interviews. Four researchers independently devised questionnaire items from this list. These were then discussed jointly, scrutinised for repetition and ambiguity, and a final set of items was agreed. This led to a final list of 78 items, which were drafted in such a way as to ask about the influence of ALS on a specific area of life over the past 2 weeks. For each question, respondents could select from a range of answers as follows: never, 0; occasionally, 1; rarely, 2; often, 3; always (or cannot do at all), 4. The face validity of the questionnaire was assessed at this stage by two patients, a regional care adviser and two neurologists. No alterations were suggested. Consequently, 75 copies of the form were sent to patients with MND, with a request to complete the questionnaire and to indicate any alterations that they would suggest. A telephone number was provided in case patients wished to telephone with comments. Few comments were made about the measure, and no single issue was consistently raised. It was therefore decided to make no alterations to the measure.

In the second stage of development of the measure, the 78-item questionnaire developed in the first stage was administered by postal survey to a sample of patients with ALS. Care advisers for regions of the Motor Neurone Disease Association Society in England, Wales and Northern Ireland were approached for assistance with recruitment. A small number of patients ($n = 25$) were not contacted in this way but volunteered to take part in the study, which had been outlined in a copy of *Thumbprint*, the UK MND Association newsletter. In total, the measure was posted to 208 patients, of whom 29 individuals did not respond, and 6 blank questionnaires were returned. Thus a response rate of 173 (83.2%) was achieved. The mean age of the sample was 62.6 years (minimum 31 years, maximum 92 years, $n = 168$). 170 respondents indicated their sex, of which 66 patients (28.2% of the total sample) were female and 104 (60.1% of the total sample) were male. The mean period since diagnosis was 37.9 months (minimum 2 months; maximum 211 months, $n = 165$). Statistical analysis of these data suggested that the measure contained five dimensions and 40 items. The statistical procedures employed at this stage are documented in full elsewhere.[20] The following areas are measured by the instrument:

- *eating and drinking* (3 items) − addresses difficulties in eating solid foods, swallowing and drinking liquids

- *communication* (7 items) − addresses a variety of problems in communicating with others (e.g. difficulties with speech, such as talking slowly, stuttering while speaking, and feeling self-conscious about speech)

- *activities of daily living/independence* (10 items) − addresses a variety of limitations in ADL (e.g. difficulties in washing oneself, dressing oneself, doing tasks around the house, as well as difficulty in writing and getting dressed)

- *mobility* (10 items) − addresses problems of mobility (e.g. difficulties in walking, standing up, going up and down stairs, and falling)

- *emotional well-being* (10 items) − addresses various emotional problems (e.g. feeling lonely, bored or depressed, a feeling of embarrassment in social situations, and feeling worried about how the disease will progress in the future).

The purpose of the measure is to indicate the extent of ill health for each domain measured. Consequently, each scale is transformed so as to have a range from 0 (the best health status as measured on the questionnaire) to 100 (the worst health status as measured on the questionnaire), with each scale being calculated as follows:

> scale score = total of raw scores of each item in the scale
> divided by maximum possible raw score of
> all items in the scale, multiplied by 100.

The correlations of items with their scale totals and the internal consistency reliability of scales (i.e. the extent to which items in a scale tap a single underlying dimension) were evaluated in order to assess the psychometric soundness of the instrument. Items were found to be highly correlated with their own scale score (corrected so as not to include the item with which it was being correlated). Internal reliability was assessed using Cronbach's alpha statistic,[21] and all of the scales were found to have very high internal consistency reliability by any standards, but particularly high reliability by the standard for group comparisons.[22,23]

Construct validity was assessed in two small-scale studies. In the first it was examined by means of correlations of scales for the ALSAQ-40 with relevant scales for the SF-36. The mobility scale of the ALSAQ-40 correlated with the physical function scale of the SF-36. The activities of daily living/independence scale of the ALSAQ-40 correlated with both the physical function scale and the role limitations due to physical problems scale of the SF-36. The emotional well-being scale of the ALSAQ-40 was found to be correlated with both the mental health and role limitations due to emotional problems scales of the SF-36. These associations had been postulated previously and give further evidence that the ALSAQ-40 provides a meaningful picture of health status.

The acceptability and construct validity of the ALSAQ was also assessed in a pilot study undertaken in a neurology clinic in the USA. Patients completed the forms without difficulty. The internal reliability of the measure was found to be comparable to that obtained in the UK samples. High correlations were found between conceptually similar domains on a clinician-completed form (the ALS-FRS) and domains of the ALSAQ. The eating and drinking domain (ALSAQ-40) correlated with speech, swallowing and breathing (ALS-FRS). Communication (ALSAQ-40) correlated with the ALS-FRS domains of speech, salivation, swallowing and breathing. ALSAQ-40 activities of daily living/independence domain scores correlated with ALS-FRS domains of writing, cutting food, dressing and hygiene, turning in bed, walking and climbing stairs. Physical mobility (ALSAQ-40) correlated with turning in bed, walking and climbing stairs. The only unexpected association was that found between emotional reactions (ALSAQ-40) and the turning in bed dimension of the ALS-FRS. However, this may be accounted for by the fact that discomfort in bed is likely to lead to poor sleep which in turn causes tiredness and fatigue, which evidence suggests is associated with poor mental health.[24]

Discussion

Research into patient-based outcome and quality of life takes a wider perspective than the purely medical model of disease that has until now dominated clinical trials and other assessments of the value of treatments. The future of treatment for ALS is beginning to show promise, and simply assessing functional ability or length of life will not provide a full insight into the impact of new treatment regimes. Subjective reports of patients will provide a far more comprehensive picture of the effects of treatment. Furthermore, a very strong case can be made for measuring carer burden and quality of life. The full potential of quality-of-life measurements will only begin to be realised when the full social and economic effects are understood. After the development and application of new disease-specific measures for ALS, the next important task will be the creation of measures to be completed by those who care for individuals with the disease.

In conclusion, it is argued that in studies of future treatments for ALS, research should systematically measure quality of life and health status. Given the limited impact that medicine can have on the prognosis of this disease at present, it is essential that treatment at the very least improves well-being and quality of life. Further validation of and experience with generic measures will increase their use by and value to the neurological community, and the application of ALS-specific outcome measures will provide important end-point measures for future trials and cohort studies.

References

1 Brooks BR (1966) Clinical epidemiology of amyotrophic lateral sclerosis. *Neurol Clin.* **14**: 399–420.

2 Leigh PN and Swash M (1995) *Motor Neuron Disease: Biology and Management.* Springer-Verlag, London.

3 Rosser R (1993) A health index and output measure. In: SR Walker and R Rosser (eds) *Quality of Life Assessment: Key Issues in the 1990s.* Kluwer, London.

4 Norris FH, Calanchini PR, Fallat RJ, Pantry S and Jewett B (1974) The administration of guanidine in amyotrophic lateral sclerosis. *Neurology.* **34**: 721–8.

5 Brooks B, Sufit R, DePaul R, Tan Y, Senjak M and Robbins J (1991) Design of clinical therapeutic trials in amyotrophic lateral sclerosis. *Adv Neurol.* **56**: 521–46.

6 Appel V, Stewart SS, Smith G and Appel SH (1987) A rating scale for amyotrophic lateral sclerosis: description and preliminary experience. *Ann Neurol.* **22**: 328–33.

7 The ALS Ciliary Neurotrophic Factor (CNTF) Treatment Study Phase I–II Study Group (1996) The Amyotrophic Lateral Sclerosis Functional Rating Scale. Assessment of

activities of daily living in patients with amyotrophic lateral sclerosis. *Arch Neurol.* **53**; 141–7.

8 Cedarbaum JM and Stambler N (1997) Performance of the Amyotrophic Lateral Sclerosis Functional Rating Scale (ALSFRS) in multicenter clinical trials. *J Neurol Sci.* **152 (Supplement 1)**: S1–9.

9 Cedarbaum JM, Stambler M and Malta E *et al.* (1999) The ALSFRS-R: a revised ALS functional rating scale that incorporates assessments of respiratory function. *J Neurol Sci.* **169**: 13–21.

10 Ware J and Sherbourne C (1992) The MOS 36-Item Short-Form Health Survey. 1. Conceptual framework and item selection. *Med Care.* **30**: 473–83.

11 Young CA, Tedman BM and Williams IR (1995) Disease progression and perceptions of health in patients with motor neurone disease. *J Neurol Sci.* **129 (Supplement)**: 50–53.

12 Shields RK, Ruhland JL, Ross MA, Saehler MM, Smith KB and Heffner ML (1998) Analysis of health-related quality of life and muscle impairment in individuals with amyotrophic lateral sclerosis using the Medical Outcome Survey and the Tufts Quantitative Neuromuscular Exam. *Arch Phys Med Rehabil.* **79**: 855–6.

13 Jenkinson C, Swash M and Fitzpatrick R for the European ALS-HPS Steering Group (1998) The European Amyotrophic Lateral Sclerosis Health Profile Study. *J Neurol Sci.* **160 (Supplement)**: 122–6.

14 Jenkinson C, Stewart-Brown S, Petersen S and Paice C (1999) Evaluation of the SF-36 Version II in the United Kingdom. *J Epidemiol Commmun Health.* **53**: 46–50.

15 Ware J, Kosinski M and Keller SD (1996) A 12-Item Short-Form Health Survey: construction of scales and preliminary tests of reliability and validity. *Med Care.* **3**: 220–23.

16 Miller RG, Anderson FA, Bradley WG *et al.* (2000) The ALS Patient Care Database: goals, design and early results. *Am Acad Neurol.* **54**: 53–7.

17 Damiano AM, Patrick DL, Guzman G *et al.* (1999) Measurement of health-related quality of life in patients with amyotrophic lateral sclerosis in clinical trials of new therapies. *Med Care.* **37**: 15–26.

18 McGuire D, Garrison L, Armon C *et al.* (1996) Relationship of the Tufts Quantitative Neuromuscular Exam (TQNE) and the Sickness Impact Profile (SIP) in measuring progression of ALS. Syntex-Synergen Neuroscience Joint Venture ALS Study Group. *Neurology.* **46**: 1442–4.

19 McGuire D, Garrison L, Armon C *et al.* (1997) A brief quality-of-life measure for ALS clinical trials based on a subset of items from the Sickness Impact Profile. The Syntex-Synergen ALS/CNTF Study Group. *J Neurol Sci.* **152 (Supplement 1)**: S18–22.

20 Jenkinson C, Fitzpatrick R, Brennan C, Bromberg M and Swash M (1999) Development and validation of a short measure of health status for individuals with amyotrophic lateral sclerosis. *J Neurol.* **246 (Supplement 3)**: 16–21.

21 Cronbach LJ (1951) Coefficient alpha and the internal structure of tests. *Psychometrika.* **16**: 297–334.

22 Nunnally JC and Bernstein IH (1994) *Psychometric Theory* (3e). McGraw Hill, New York.

23 Ware JE, Kosinski M and Keller SD (1994) *SF-36 Physical and Mental Health Summary Scales. A User's Manual.* The Health Institute, New England Medical Center, Boston, MA.

24 Walker EA, Katon WJ and Jemalka RP (1993) Psychiatric disorders and medical care utilisation among people in the general population who report fatigue. *J Gen Intern Med.* **8**: 436–40.

9
The translation and cross-cultural adaptation of quality-of-life measures

Alyson Grove, Patricia Grey Amante, Paul Quarterman and Diane Wild

Introduction

It is becoming increasingly common for measures of quality of life to be included in studies evaluating neurological diseases or treatments. There are now a number of questionnaires available which have been developed specifically for patients with neurological diseases.[1] With the increasing internationalisation of trials and other studies, demand is increasing for quality-of-life measures which are available for use across cultures.[2–5]

It is important therefore to ensure that an instrument developed in one culture is valid in another. The achievement of cross-cultural comparability requires attention to the following issues:

- the content of the questionnaire and its conceptual basis
- the method of translation
- the testing and comparison of reliability, validity, responsiveness and effect size within each country or culture.

With demand increasing throughout the world for quality-of-life measures that are available in several languages and which are also equally appropriate for use in different cultures, attention to these issues in research is becoming increasingly important. The rising demand is due in part to the development of global perspectives on health and healthcare. Clinical trials are increasingly international, resulting in the need to aggregate data across sample populations from different countries. Provision and regulation of healthcare, although still primarily a national responsibility, are affected by transnational agreements on provider licensing and certification, standards of care, and applications of medical technology. The approval process and market for treatments, particularly pharmaceuticals, are becoming more international. This global perspective has prompted the development of quality-of-life measures in which data can be aggregated across different cultures.

Interest in cross-cultural quality-of-life measures is furthered by the desire to strengthen causal inference in the evaluation of treatments. As diagnostic criteria become more international, treatment is becoming more standardised in different cultures, thus prompting attempts to compare outcomes of treatment in different cultural settings, particularly using randomised clinical trials. Causal inference and external validity may be strengthened if the same effect is found cross-culturally. Finally, there is a growing interest in comparing different geographical regions, different social and physical environments, and different populations in order to identify optimal social and health policies, to monitor trends, and to make political claims.

The move towards development of cross-culturally applied measures of quality of life is tempered by the recognition that wide differences exist in the cultural notions of health and illness, and in how different populations react to what is presumably the same biological condition. As cultural anthropologists demonstrate repeatedly, a person's conception of what constitutes 'disease' or 'health' can depend on his or her cultural traditions. Language and group mores, as well as more individual characteristics such as age, educational level and income, can also have an impact.[6,7] Consequently, comparisons cannot be made without considering the cross-cultural content of measures, the cultural meaning of different domains, the translation of measures from one language to another, and the cross-cultural testing of measurement properties, all of which are important considerations in assessing quality of life.

Issues in cross-cultural research

To the extent that functional status – defined as activities such as walking, sleeping, eating and working – is found in every culture, it seems reasonable that an instrument assessing function could produce valid cross-cultural results. There appears to be a core set of specific behaviours that transfer readily between cultures. Symptoms may also be described similarly in different cultures. Subjective reactions to symptoms and health conditions – that is, the value assigned to health and living conditions, the relative importance of different states, standards of behaviour, and the meaning of different health states – may show more cultural variation. These subjective perceptions, particularly values and preferences for health, define quality of life.[2,8] The extent to which functional status and broader quality-of-life domains have universal definitions and meaning across cultures is both a theoretical and an empirical question.

Cross-cultural comparability also seems plausible to the extent that biology and its consequences are something which all people tend to share, with some exceptions. Similarly, because the social roles of , for example, parent, worker and student are comparable, they provide opportunities to evaluate function cross-culturally. However, the inclusion of more culturally specific domains (or the necessary exclusion of others), as well as variation in the natural history of disease, are barriers to the design of valid cross-cultural instruments. It may be unclear whether differences in quality-of-life scores between cultures should be attributed to variation in the biological response, the cultural setting, the psychosocial constructs used in measurement, or the measurement process itself.

What is meant by the term 'cross-cultural'? For many parts of the world, 'cross-cultural' cannot be equated with 'cross-national', because of the ethnic diversity that exists within national boundaries. The assumption of cultural comparability in measures derived from a single sample in a country may therefore be invalid. In practice, however, the early development of a measure may begin with a single sample representing a nation, with extensions to different groups at a later date. How many cultures and what scope of cultural variation are necessary to test the cross-cultural validity of a quality-of-life instrument? At the very minimum, it seems that the unqualified use of the phrase 'cross-culturally valid' is not particularly informative. However, cultural and linguistic differences can have a significant effect on the way in which individuals perceive their experiences of health and illness,[9] and are therefore critically important.

Between language versions, linguistic differences are fairly obvious, but cultural differences are less easy to determine. Although the term 'culture' is frequently referred to as an important concept throughout the social sciences, there does not appear to be a single accepted definition of the concept. However, from cultural anthropology we find that culture includes 'learned and shared ways of interpreting the world and interacting in society',[10] so that it essentially gives individuals within that society a way to think about what is acceptable or unacceptable behaviour, for example, or what is important or unimportant in life. Thus we cannot escape from the idea that an individual's perceptions or attitudes towards their own quality of life are, at least to some extent, 'culture bound', and while cultural relativism suggests that there are some basics to human existence which are universally accepted as such, there are no set standards of quality of life which can similarly be applied equally to all cultures.[10]

An important issue in trying to define 'culture' and what impact it has on people's quality of life is at the personal level of social comparison,[11] based on Festinger's social comparison theory.[12] Festinger suggested that people compare themselves with others when there is no objective basis for defining their situation or circumstances, and that the people with whom they choose to compare themselves are people who are similar to them. Although he does not actually use the term 'social comparison', Sartorius discussed this type of theory in terms of health and quality of life, and proposed that comparisons about illness are made at three levels:[13,14]

- intrapersonal – where people make comparisons with their own experience, such as what they would like their health to be, and the best and worst health they have ever experienced

- interpersonal – where people make comparisons with other people's experiences (either other people with the same illness, people in their own social group or people in other social groups)

- sociocultural – where people make comparisons with society's expectations of how they should behave or react to their illness.

In a study of social comparisons in quality-of-life perception, Skevington[11] collected data via focus groups with patients with arthritic disease. The patients discussed the different factors that might have an influence on their quality of life and their expectations about their future. These were considered against the same data from a group of 'healthy' individuals. The data were examined for the presence of the three types of comparisons outlined by Sartorius.[13,14] The results of the discussions showed that quality of life was mostly discussed in terms of social comparison, because people did not seem to have an objective basis for defining quality of life. Many of the patients discussed their quality of life in intrapersonal terms, referring mainly to things they could no longer do, etc. Interpersonal comparisons were also used, with references made to the age and health of others in an attempt to describe their own situation. There were discussions which centred around sociocultural comparisons, with references to what society thought about them and their illness. In some instances, people used a combination of two of these types of comparisons. Thus social comparisons are clearly used in people's understanding and perceptions of their quality of life. These types of comparisons are essentially culture bound, which means that a questionnaire developed within one culture which has 'tapped into' the perceptions of that one society must, as a matter of course, be used with caution in other societies or cultures. This must be kept in mind during the translation and cultural validation process.

Sechrest *et al.* describe four main types of problems which may be encountered in cross-cultural research.[15]

- Participants in the study need to be given some kind of explanation of why they are being asked to participate in the study (i.e. a study rationale), which should be the same for each patient in all countries, yet there seems to be no reference to this in most multinational research papers, either as a problem or as an element of the research process.

- The quality of the translation of instructions for participants also seems to be largely assumed, as very little of this process is ever discussed in the reporting of cross-cultural research studies.

- Questions need to be phrased so that they are comparable in different languages. This is a well-recognised issue, but it still causes many difficulties in establishing a new translation of an existing measure. Most commonly, the words used are too sophisticated for the target population, or colloquial expressions are used which in themselves have no relevance to a different culture.

- Translating responses to open-ended questions can also prove difficult, as this may require the translation of the coding directions, or trusting that bilingual scorers understand the items in the way that they were intended by the developer. Of course, inter-rater reliability can also be a problem, especially when the 'raters' come from different countries.

There are three questions about quality of life which may be asked in relation to any given culture. First, what is quality of life in that national context? Secondly, how are quality-of-life questions asked? Thirdly, what do any observed changes in quality of life actually mean for the people concerned?[16]

Cella *et al.*[17] have also outlined a number of considerations that should be raised when planning to include a quality-of-life assessment in a clinical trial. These include the natural history of the disease or condition (which may not change very much between cultures), the characteristics of the population (which may show differences between different cultures), the treatment under consideration (which is likely to be the same in clinical trials) and the function of the trial organisation (which may be centred in one country for all international sites, or it may be local).

Hunt[9] suggests a 'new approach' to cross-cultural adaptation, which is based on the 'needs-based model'. The model was designed with the idea that it may be able to overcome some of the culturally linked issues that make cross-cultural adaptation so difficult. Its approach is that quality of life is not about what a person is able to do in a functional sense, but rather it concerns a person's ability to fulfil or satisfy their basic human needs for such things as social interaction, affection, etc.[18] It is thought that this approach minimises cultural specificity and ambiguity.[9]

However, with such demand for the production of measures which can be used in multinational research studies, there is a constant request for the production of new language versions of the existing measures, which inevitably leads to the translation of the existing measures.

Translation

The main aim of the translation process is to establish conceptual and semantic equivalence across all language versions. Conceptual equivalence refers to whether the same concept exists in another language or culture. Semantic equivalence refers to whether the same linguistic expression exists in another language or culture. Where conceptual and semantic equivalence are both present, the items in a cross-cultural measure are identical across languages. If the concept exists but not the expression, then the solution is to change the expression in the new language. If the expression exists but not the concept, then the item is culturally specific. If neither the concept nor the expression is present, then it is impossible to translate the item into the other language.[9] This is because vocabulary itself is more than just words. It has a cultural context which helps to give the words specific meanings or connotations.[19] This is what essentially makes translation difficult,[20] but it also therefore follows that the items or measures which are used successfully after translation into other languages depend on the extent to which the different cultures for which they have been translated have an overlap or are similar to the original culture in which the item or measure was developed.[21]

This is an interesting point, as equivalence of language may often be used as a justification for the belief that a measure developed in one country (e.g. the USA) is likely to work well in another country (e.g. the UK), whereas culturally the UK is likely to be closer in experience to European countries which do not share English as the main language.[19] It may even be the case that there are significant differences between the cultural influences on different population groups within the same country (e.g. the USA), which should be similarly respected.[22] In addition, the structure of the instrument itself may prove problematic in some countries where patients may not be accustomed to the use of self-completion forms as a means of conveying information. This kind of information elicitation is very common in the USA and the UK in particular, as well as throughout most of the Western world, but other countries may not have the experience of knowing how to respond to a list of questions. Hunt demonstrates this in her description of the attempt to adapt the Nottingham Health Profile into Arabic for Egypt, where some of the items were met with embarrassment and disgust.[23] Thus theoretical and conceptual issues which are not generally found in research within a single country will appear at various stages of the research process when cross-cultural validity is sought.[24] Attention should therefore be paid not only to issues such as the way in which questions are worded or how measures are translated, but also to the construct validity of the measures themselves.[25]

In 1994, Guillemin et al. proposed a set of guidelines specifically for cross-cultural adaptation of quality-of-life measures.[26] They suggested that the aim of cross-cultural adaptation should be to maintain the content and face validity of the original measure by establishing semantic, idiomatic, experiential and conceptual equivalence. This can be achieved by using forward and backward translation methods, review by a committee, pilot testing and weighting the scores for the target culture, where this is relevant. However, Guillemin et al. did not provide definitions of these terms, or describe the basis for deciding when it is relevant to weight the scores, or even how to weight them.

A more useful approach to developing and evaluating constructs (such as quality-of-life measures) for use cross-nationally was proposed by Hui and Triandis.[27] They suggested that there were four dimensions of equivalence which should be assessed.

1   *Conceptual or functional equivalence* – whether a construct that has meaning in one culture can also be meaningfully discussed in another culture.

2   *Construct equivalence* – whether the same methods are used to elicit information in the different cultural groups, and whether the methods themselves are equally meaningful in those cultures.

3 *Item equivalence* – whether the construct can be measured by the same instrument in different cultures. This assumes that the two previous types of equivalence already exist, and it implies that each of the items in a measure should mean the same thing to each respondent in all cultures. It is possible that a lack of item equivalence can be corrected or improved by rigorous translation methods, but of course this can only be true if an instrument has conceptual equivalence.

4 *Scalar equivalence* – whether an instrument is able to categorise different groups (e.g. in terms of degree of illness) in a similar way regardless of culture. This type of equivalence is the most difficult to achieve.

No one of these types of equivalence can be cited as sufficient evidence for the existence of cross-cultural equivalence. The more abstract types must be in place for more specific types of equivalence to be possible.

The guidelines and terminology used in the quality-of-life field to describe these types of equivalence have been criticised by Herdman *et al.*,[28] who say that there is a lack of clear definition of 'equivalence', and that the field therefore lacks a theoretical framework to establish this equivalence. It is true, of course, that most multinational drug trials choose an existing quality-of-life measure and therefore opt to translate it into the other languages that they require. This demand has resulted in a proliferation of papers on methodology and on defining the different types of 'equivalence', many of which contradict one another.

A variety of health status measures is used, including the basic calculation of morbidity and mortality statistics, physical symptom measures, diagnostic instruments, and a whole range of instruments to measure physical and psychological functioning and impairment. Many of these measures were developed for specific settings, and are used exclusively in that context. Often such measures are translated into another language and used in another country without any consideration being given to the data-pooling implications of such a step. The development of different language versions of an instrument facilitates the comparison of results from different countries only when it is done in a rigorous manner. This means not only that basic methodological principles are adhered to, but also that consideration is given to the cultural differences that exist between different countries.[29] These will include basic elements such as cultural concepts of health and illness, literacy and reading levels, and taboo or sensitive subjects.

The problems of producing translations of health status measures which have international validity are not unique — they are similar to the types of problems encountered by any scientific attempt to work cross-culturally with a standard measurement,[30] as cross-cultural stability in the social sciences in particular is not necessarily present. This is because the attitudes and values against which people judge their own health perceptions are culturally diverse.[7,31]

It is well documented, if not so well practised, that translating instruments into another language does not simply require the rewriting of the words into the new language.[22] A 'good' translation also requires the consideration of psychological, linguistic and cultural factors.[32] As Van de Vijver and Tanzer point out,[33] there are two main approaches to developing a translation. One is the forward–backward translation approach, whereby the forward translation is checked for accuracy against the back translation, and the other is the committee approach, in which the items are translated by a group of people with different areas of expertise (e.g. cultural, linguistic or psychological). The problem with the forward–backward translation approach is that, although items can be translated into the target language with relative ease, with the back translation indicating the accuracy of the translation, there is no means of detecting any potential psychological difficulties. A clear example of good linguistic equivalence but a lack of psychological equivalence was cited by Hambleton,[32] who found that the English item

'Where is a bird with webbed feet most likely to live?' had been translated into Swedish as 'Where is a bird with swimming feet most likely to live?', which gives the respondent a much stronger clue to the answer. This type of problem is more likely to be avoided with the committee translation approach.

Another option is to use the adaptation approach, which gives greater flexibility as to which items should not be included in a new translation, and whether any items need to be added. This approach was used by Spielberger et al.[34] in the development of the State–Trait Anxiety Inventory (STAI), of which more than 40 language versions exist. These versions are not literal translations of the original language, but are adapted so that the underlying constructs, in this case state and trait anxiety, are measured in a satisfactory way by each language version.[35]

However, in some instances the instrument has to be changed so much that the result is virtually a new measure. This option is called 'assembly', and is particularly relevant when a construct bias due to different levels of appropriateness of items within different cultures is present. A good example of this type of difficulty is discussed by Church,[36] who argues that Western culture as a whole does not encompass the personality constructs found in the Filipino culture. Similarly, Cheung et al.[37] argue that adapting a Western personality measure for use in a Chinese culture could not capture all of the relevant dimensions of personality found in that culture.

A particular difficulty in the whole translation process arises from the tight deadlines which must often be adhered to during the production of new language versions of existing measures. The temptation in these circumstances is to conduct the translation work for a variety of languages in one country, using bilingual translators, rather than having in-country translators involved in the process. This has been deemed a satisfactory approach,[38] provided that a final pilot test is carried out among the target population.

However, in 1997, the Medical Outcomes Trust (MOT) introduced 'New Translation Criteria',[39] which set out the framework within which the translation of quality-of-life measures should be undertaken. They suggest that initially any instrument which is to undergo a translation process should be reviewed by the Scientific Advisory Committee and approved by the MOT, and then the following 'minimal translation criteria' should be fulfilled:

- two independent forward translations of the instrument, for which documented evidence is available

- one back translation of the instrument, for which documented evidence is also available

- a detailed description of the translation process must be available, including information about the population involved in the debriefing process and, where possible, information about the qualifications of the translators used to do the translation work.

Finally, all of the above information, including details of any modifications made to the translation during the process, must be documented and made available.

This method avoids, to some extent, the specific psychological and cultural difficulties outlined earlier, as it advocates testing the translated measure within the target population group. However, sensitivity to and respect for cultural differences should be maintained at each stage of the process. Essentially, this requires that the forward translation work be done at least partly in the country concerned.

There are a number of important limitations to this approach.[40]

- The original (usually English) wording is likely to have problems which, in an attempt to ensure that new translations do not stray very far from the original language, tend to be perpetuated throughout any subsequent translated versions.

- Particular items which work perfectly well in the original language may simply not translate well into other languages, so that some items end up being poorly worded in the target language simply because they remain close to the original.

- Some items are not really translatable at all, or are simply nonsensical within the context of the target culture.

- Items in a measure which was developed in one country may have been included because of their salience to that population, whereas the same items address issues which are completely irrelevant to other cultures. Similarly, the most important issues in the new culture may be missing from the original questionnaire.

- Broadly speaking, these limitations perpetuate the idea that the only issues which are of any real importance in any given situation are those which affect the middle-class English speaker (most often American).

So how can we overcome these problems? The basic focus of any research of this kind should be what one is actually trying to measure — the essence of what is being studied, regardless of the native tongue in which one is working. Once the main aim is clear, an instrument which meets these requirements must be found. Most often, of course, this instrument will exist for English-speakers but not for anyone else. This is where the difficulties arise. How do we find out the same information from other populations? The new approach, which is suggested by Guyatt,[40] is that the existing (usually English) version be used simply as a template and guide for subsequent versions. Thus it should immediately be acknowledged that:

1   the original version has problems which the new 'translations' may be able to improve on rather than simply duplicate

2   the target population is likely to have different issues within the area of interest to those raised by the population in which the measure was developed, some of the issues included may not be familiar to the target population, and where there are issues that are important to both groups, the means of responding may not apply equally to both groups.

If all of these factors were taken into consideration at the outset, anyone attempting to produce a new language version of an existing questionnaire would not have as their primary aim the exact replication of the original version using a different language.

There are three levels of options for avoiding this methodology.

No expense spared

If time and money were irrelevant, the best approach would be to replicate the entire process which was used to develop the original measure in each of the target populations. This would therefore include item generation and item reduction. The resulting measure(s) may closely mirror the original version, but may also be entirely different.

The cheap version

With limited resources, one might assume that the basic structure and content of the original language version of the existing instrument have some relevance for measuring that health area in the target population, and thus set out on the usual path of translation. However, when translators find what they consider to be deficiencies in the original version, they should be encouraged to improve on the language they are given, provided that they can argue their case effectively. Thus in the case of items which simply do not translate well, new items may be substituted from other questionnaires which already exist in the target language, or new items may be added for original items that cannot be translated at all. Then, in the pilot-testing phase, highly problematic or irrelevant questions should be deleted, and issues which are important to the target group which were not originally included should be added to fill these omissions.

The 'in-between' version

This is based on using an original version along the same lines as described for the 'cheap version' above, but with the addition of an intermediate step. The assumptions one might make are that the domains included in the original version are likely to be important to the target population, and that the methods used to produce the items and their corresponding response options will work in the target population. The important new step, however, is that a translation of the original version is taken into focus groups and the appropriateness of the domains, items and response options is challenged within the context of the target language/culture/population. Thus again the new language version of the instrument may be very similar to the original, but it could also be very different.

The two major difficulties with this approach are that aggregating results across countries is very difficult, and it also has to be questioned what conclusions can be drawn from two questionnaires which look so very different.

Psychometric testing

Culture can influence a given psychological measure in two ways.[41]

1   It can affect the pattern of the relationships between items (the patterning effect). For example, where the correlation between two items in one culture is positive, it may be negative in another, which would mean that the relationship between the items is culture-specific. Where correlations between items in different cultures are similar, the relationships between items can be said to be the same across cultures.

2   It can affect the position of the responses given by individuals to different items (the positioning effect). For example, the correlation between two items may be the same, but one culture group may have much higher scores than the other. This would mean that if the responses were plotted on a graph, the two groups of responses would appear in different locations. Similarly, the two groups may have different correlations between two items, but when plotted on a graph they may appear at a similar location.

Paunonen and Ashton[42] reviewed six structured personality questionnaires and outlined five psychometric properties which, if 'equivalent', indicate that the measure may be suitable for use in different cultures. These are the scale mean, variance, reliability, criterion validity and factorial structure. However, concern has been expressed about the extent to which finding a similar factor structure for the same measure in different cultures 'proves' that the theoretical structure of the measure and responses to individual items are also equivalent across those culture groups. Byrne and Campbell[43] explored the extent to which item scores on a measure can vary across cultures, despite finding that measure to have an 'excellent fit' to a specified factor structure when tested separately in each cultural group, as they found with the Beck Depression Inventory (BDI)[44] when it was used on adolescents in Bulgaria, Canada and Sweden.

It cannot be assumed therefore that a questionnaire, however extensively it is tested in the country of origin, will be valid and reliable once it has been translated. No instrument for the assessment of psychological states or subjective perceptions is culture free. In each instance the validity and other characteristics of the instrument must be assessed within the culture of application. In particular, attention must be paid to the following properties.

Reliability

Reliability is a generic term that refers to the stability and equivalence of repeated measures of the same concept. Reliability coefficients estimate the proportion of observed error that can be considered to be 'true' as opposed to 'random'.[45] In order to be able to discriminate between people in cross-sectional studies, internal consistency reliability is important, using the coefficient 'alpha'. This gives the correlation between items in an instrument. The value of alpha will be higher when items included in the measure of a particular concept or domain have a high average correlation between responses to all possible combinations of items in that domain. In longitudinal investigations where change over time is assessed, reproducibility, stability and responsiveness are important for distinguishing between those who remain stable and those who experience change. In cross-cultural validation studies, assessment of internal consistency is straightforward. The alpha coefficient can be calculated on all component domains of the instrument. The higher the coefficient, the better the internal consistency of the measure. An acceptable level of alpha for quality-of-life measures has been defined as ≥ 0.70.[4] In most cases this level will be relatively easy to achieve if multiple items are generated and tested for each quality-of-life domain.

Reproducibility or test–retest reliability refers to the correlation between responses to the same items administered to the same respondents at different times. If something is highly variable by nature, it is difficult to observe whether differences in repeated measures are caused by chance in the observed phenomenon or by non-reproducible observations. With quality-of-life measures, reproducibility is preferably measured using the interclass correlation coefficient, which corrects for agreement that would be expected simply by chance.[46] Reproducibility can be tested in each cross-cultural setting by administering the quality-of-life measure at an interval long enough to avoid recall of previous answers and test learning, but short enough for the actual states or perceptions to be likely to remain the same.

Validity

Techniques for assessing validity are more limited. Validity is a more emotionally charged term than reliability, because conceptions vary widely as to how investigators might be led astray when drawing conclusions from the data. The three commonest approaches to assessing validity are content validity, criterion validity and construct validity.

Content validity

This refers to whether a particular measure adequately represents the domain or universe of content that it is supposed to measure. Ware[47] recommends including physical, mental, social and perpetual health as a minimum standard for content in comprehensive generic measures of health-related quality of life. Content validity can be assessed using other methods. For example, Aday[48] suggests reviewing the literature and ensuring that at least one item is represented on the questionnaire for each domain identified. Another method for ensuring content validity involves factor analysis. The latter can serve many purposes, including determining the latent variable structure underlying a set of items, providing a means of explaining variation between many original variables, and defining the substantive content or meaning of the factors.[49] If a set of items tested in different languages and cultures demonstrates a similar factor structure, this similarity is an indication of shared core meaning and organisation of meaning for the items under investigation. Countries can be compared on the items that contribute to the shared content as well as those that do not. Some items may be country or culture specific. For example, similarity of the factor structure in UK and French populations was accepted as evidence of validity for a quality-of-life scale for older adults.[50] A lack of comparable factor structure has also been used to determine a lack of validity in a quality-of-life scale with regard to community satisfaction. Although the notion of community appears to have been understood by both UK and American participants, the meaning of the items differed substantially.[51] Whilst this kind of analysis has been used by investigators to suggest that an instrument is cross-culturally valid, because the underlying 'factor structure' is similar for the cultural groups studied, it is important to note that factor analysis can only confirm those domains that have been put forward for confirmation. An instrument developed in one country could easily miss important domains in another, and this would not be revealed in factor analysis. A further method of establishing content validity during the development phase of a quality-of-life measure is based on the 'needs-based model', which is a theoretical model developed by Hunt and McKenna.[18] In the model, both conceptual and semantic equivalence are required before an item can be included in a cross-cultural instrument. This approach differs greatly from all others in that it does not involve translation of an existing instrument developed in just one country. Rather, it involves the concurrent development of an instrument that is intended for cross-cultural application from its inception. In this approach, patient interviews are used for item generation and to assess the content validity of the instrument, often in the form of cognitive interviews. These include concurrent 'think-aloud' responses to items, retrospective think-aloud responses, focused interviews and paraphrasing.[52]

Criterion validity

This refers to the correspondence between a proposed measure and another measure of the same phenomenon regarded as a gold standard. This is the most prized type of validity. However, no 'gold standard' exists for most behavioural and perception-based quality-of-life measures. Some investigators suggest adopting an existing measure as the gold standard against which to compare other measures. However, there is no basis for identifying a single measure that can serve as such a criterion.

Construct validity

This refers to the use of theory to guide the comparison of measures or groups to assess the validity of measure. The main method used to provide evidence of construct validity is to compare one measure with another. This involves specifying the factors, or constructs, that account for variance in the proposed measures as well as the postulated relationships between them. Hypotheses are related regarding the direction and, if possible, the strength of relationships that might be expected. Validity is supported when the associations are consistent with prior hypotheses. The construct validity of some generic health status measures has been established, although no general theory of expected differences has emerged.[2] Moreover, cross-cultural attempts to assess construct validity are usually impossible because of the lack of parallel instruments available in all cultures. Consequently, validity is often tested uniquely in each country.[53]

Responsiveness

The ability of an instrument to detect small but important changes can be referred to as its responsiveness,[54] although some investigators prefer to consider this a type of validity for assessing change. Advance knowledge of a measure's responsiveness aids in selecting measures, permits accurate estimation of sample size to ensure sufficient statistical power, and assists in prioritising or reducing the number of end-points to be assessed.

Population- or condition-specific measures can be more responsive than generic measures, because they tap domains of particular interest to individuals with the condition, whereby small changes may be more easily detected. For a measure to detect subtle but important changes, scores must be stable among individuals who are stable (reproducible), and changing among individuals who experience actual change, however slight that change may be. Various methods are available for measuring the responsiveness of an instrument, the commonest probably being to compare instrument scores before and after treatment of known efficacy. In this case, an improvement in scores would be evidence of responsiveness as evaluated using the paired t-test statistic for within-subject changes. Alternatively, a measure of responsiveness which is particularly applied to diagnostic technologies is the receiver operating characteristic (ROC) curve, where changes on a health status instrument are viewed as diagnostic tests for patient improvement. Using this measure, the investigator can seek to distinguish between those who improve and those who do not.[46] Another method is to calculate 'effect size'.

Effect size interpretation

Effect size is an estimate of change in quality fo life. Effect sizes translate the before-and-after changes into a standardised statistic to account for within-subject and between-subject variation. Effect sizes for generic measures are usually established over a long period of using the measure, resulting in a consensus on what constitutes a significant change score or effect size. In contrast, the meaning of effect size for condition-specific instruments must be determined as part of its development process, often with limited data. Cross-cultural interpretation of effect sizes will depend on the comparability of standards for interpretation. For example, life events may not have similar cultural meaning, and could prove difficult to use when interpreting effect sizes observed in several different countries. Global ratings of change could be influenced by cultural differences in the 'anchoring' of changes, in that cultures may not discriminate between small, medium and large changes in the same way. Relating changes in a quality-of-life measure to changes in clinical status, and using global ratings of change from the patients themselves, are most likely to achieve cross-cultural comparability in understanding of effect sizes.

Item response theory

Item response theory (IRT)[55–57] is an increasingly popular way to examine and test a measure's item and scalar equivalence cross-culturally.[27] This method uses item parameters that are derived from within the measure itself, which helps to avoid the potential difficulty of establishing neutral external criteria against which to test a measure. It is based on two primary assumptions – that all of the items in the measure are related to a single concept or trait, and that the measure has 'local independence' (i.e. given that two people have the same level of the construct being measured, one person's response to any one item is not predictive of the other person's response to any other item within the measure). If these two assumptions are true of a measure, a person's performance on the whole test can be predicted by a certain set of factors, and the relationship between their performance on any one of the items and the underlying trait itself can be described by an item characteristic curve (ICC).[58] Using statistical tests developed for the purpose,[59] differences between ICCs can be used to explore the (lack of) equivalence of an item or scale between different cultures. For example, it has recently been used in a cross-cultural comparison of the scaling of the Danish, German, Italian, Dutch, Swedish, UK and US English language versions of the SF-36,[60] to show strong scale congruence across these seven countries.

Conclusions

Cross-cultural validation of quality-of-life measures is an on-going process of repeated application of theory and measurement. The most desirable method of validation is to approach the instrument developer with the goal of cross-cultural comparability in mind. Measures that have been developed simultaneously in different cultures have the advantage of identifying as early as possible those domains and items that are more or less valid in a particular culture or population. Translation of instruments that have been developed in one culture for use in another is more common, most often because of the time and resources necessary to develop measures simultaneously in different cultures. However, the danger of translation is that the conceptual structure and domains contained in the instrument may not be sufficiently comprehensive for all cultures in which the measure is to be used.

Once translated or developed simultaneously, the next challenge is to test the reproducibility, validity and responsiveness of the instrument in each culture. It is important that the methodology for assessment is standardised across cultures as much as possible. In addition to these methodological barriers, practical challenges include commitment of sufficient resources, and frequent communication between investigators. Recruitment of comparable samples of individuals on whom to test quality-of-life measures in each country is also a major challenge.

Overcoming the conceptual, methodological and practical barriers to cross-cultural validation will require a higher level of co-operation and co-ordination of investigative sites in the different countries participating in instrument development. The achievement of conceptual and semantic equivalence and improvement of standardisation of validation procedures requires agreement on field test protocols, adherence to these protocols, and frequent communication between sites concerning problems and solutions. A wider range of populations representing different subgroups of national populations needs to be included in validation studies. Such studies are expensive, and the development of cross-culturally valid instruments requires considerable investment on the part of the study sponsors. However, such investment will be necessary in order to achieve the standardisation of measurement procedures and comparability and interpretation of outcomes.

As the development of cross-cultural measures of quality of life becomes more specialised, the expertise ensuring the reliability, validity and responsiveness of these measures will improve. The use of these measures will aid the quest for information that is relevant and informative to cultures all over the world.

References

1   Wilson RS, Goetz CG and Stebbins GT (1996) Neurologic illness. In: B Spilker (ed.) *Quality of Life and Pharmacoeconomics in Clinical Trials.* Lippincott-Raven, New York.

2   Patrick DL and Erikson P (1993) *Health Status and Health Policy: Allocating Resources to Health Care.* Oxford University Press, New York.

3   Spilker B, Molinek FR, Johnston KA, Simpson RL Jr and Tilson HH (1990) Quality of life biography and indexes. *Med Care.* **28 (Supplement 12)**: DS1–77.

4   Stewart AL and Ware JE (eds) (1992) *Measuring Functioning and Well-Being: the Medical Outcomes Study Approach.* Duke University Press, London and Durham, North Carolina.

5 Walker SR and Rosser RH (eds) (1992) *Quality of Life Assessment: Key Issues in the 1990s.* Kluwer Academic Publishers, Dordrecht.

6 Fabrega H (1974) *Disease and Social Behavior: An Interdisciplinary Perspective.* Institute of Technology Press, Cambridge, MA.

7 Kleinman A, Eisenberg L and Good B (1978) Culture, illness and care: clinical lessons from anthropologic and cross-cultural research. *Ann Intern Med.* **88**: 251–8.

8 World Health Organization Quality-of-Life Group (1993) Study protocol for the World Health Organization project to develop a Quality-of-Life Instrument (WHOQOL). *Qual Life Res.* **2**: 153–9.

9 Hunt SM (1993) Cross-cultural comparability of quality-of-life measures. *Drug Inform J.* **27**: 395–400.

10 Campos SS and Johnson TM (1990) Cultural considerations. In: B Spilker (ed.) *Quality of Life Assessments in Clinical Trials.* Raven Press, New York.

11 Skevington SM (1994) Social comparisons in cross-cultural quality-of-life assessment. *Int J Ment Health.* **23**: 29–47.

12 Festinger L (1954) A theory of social comparison processes. *Hum Relations.* **7**: 117–40.

13 Sartorius N (1987) Cross-cultural comparisons of data about quality of life: a sample of issues. In: NK Aaronson and J Backmann (eds) *The Quality of Life of Cancer Patients.* Raven Press, New York.

14 Sartorius N (1991) Quality of life. In: B Vrhovac, I Bakran, M Granić, B Jakšić, B Labar and B Vucelić (eds) *Interna Medicina.* Naprijed, Zagreb.

15 Sechrest L, Fay TL and Hafeez Zaidi SM (1972) Problems of translation in cross-cultural research. *J Cross-Cult Res.* **3**: 41–56.

16 Bullinger M, Anderson R, Cella D and Aaronson N (1993) Developing and evaluating cross-cultural instruments from minimum requirements to optimal models. *Qual Life Res.* **2**: 451–9.

17 Cella DF, Wiklund I, Shumaker SA and Aaronson NK (1993) Integrating health-related quality of life into cross-national clinical trials. *Qual Life Res.* **2**: 433–40.

18 Hunt SM and McKenna S (1992) The QLDS: a scale for the measurement of quality of life in depression. *Health Policy.* **22**: 307–19.

19 Hunt SM, Alonso J, Bucquet D, Niero M, Wiklund I and McKenna S (1991) Cross-cultural adaptation of health measures. *Health Policy.* **19**: 33–44.

20 Mills CW (1939) Language, logic and culture. In: I Horowitz (ed.) *Power, Politics and People.* Ballantine, New York.

21 Kluckhorn F and Strodtbeck F (1961) *Variations in Value Orientations.* Row, Peterson, Evanston, IL.

22 Geisinger KF (1994) Cross-cultural normative assessment: translation and adaptation issues influencing the normative interpretation of assessment instruments. *Psychol Assess.* **6**: 304–12.

23 Hunt SM (1986) Cross-cultural issues in the use of socio-medical indicators. *Health Policy.* **6**: 146–58.

24 Bice TW and Kalimo E (1971) Comparisons of health-related attitudes: a cross-national, factor analytic study. *Soc Sci Med.* **5**: 283–318.

25 Scheuch EK (1968) The cross-cultural use of sample surveys: problems of comparability. In: S Rokkan (ed.) *Comparative Research Across Cultures and Nations.* Mouton, Paris.

26 Guillemin F, Bombardier C and Beaton D (1994) Guidelines for the cross-cultural adaptation of health-related quality of life measures. *Qual Life Res.* **3**: 42.

27 Hui CH and Triandis HC (1985) Measurement in cross-cultural psychology: a review and comparison of strategies. *J Cross-Cult Psychol.* **16**: 131–52.

28 Herdman M, Fox-Rushby J and Badia X (1997) 'Equivalence' and the translation and adaptation of health-related quality of life questionnaires. *Qual Life Res.* **6**: 237–47.

29 Sartorius N and Kuyken W (1994) Translation of health status instruments. In: J Orley and W Kuyken (eds) *Quality*

of Life Assessment: International Perspectives. Springer-Verlag, Berlin.

30 Bullinger M (1994) Ensuring international equivalence of quality of life measures: problems and approaches to solutions. In: J Orley and W Kuyken (eds) *Quality of Life Assessment: International Perspectives.* Springer-Verlag, Berlin.

31 Dressler WW, Vieteri FE, Chavez A, Greel GAC and Santos JE (1991) Comparative research in social epidemiology: measurement issues. *Ethnicity Dis.* **1**: 379–93.

32 Hambleton RK (1994) Guidelines for adapting educational and psychological tests: a progress report. *Eur J Psychol Assess.* **10**: 229–35.

33 Van de Vijver F and Tanzer NK (1997) Bias and equivalence in cross-cultural assessment: an overview. *Eur Rev Appl Psychol.* **47**: 263–79.

34 Spielberger CD, Gorsuch RL and Lushene R (1970) *Manual for the State–Trait Anxiety Inventory.* Consulting Psychologists Press, Palo Alto, CA.

35 Laux L, Glanzmann P, Schaffner P and Spielberger CD (1981) *The German Adaptation of the State–Trait Anxiety Inventory. Theoretical Background and Manual.* Beltz Test, Weinheim.

36 Church TA (1987) Personality research in a non-Western setting: the Philippines. *Psychol Bull.* **102**: 272–92.

37 Cheung FM, Leung K, Fan RM, Song WZ, Zhang JX and Chang JP (1996) Development of the Chinese Personality Assessment Inventory. *J Cross-Cult Psychol.* **27**: 181–99.

38 Mathias SD, Fifer SK and Patrick DL (1994) Rapid translation of quality of life measures for international clinical trials: avoiding errors in the minimalist approach. *Qual Life Res.* **3**: 403–12.

39 Medical Outcomes Trust (1997) Trust introduces new translation criteria. *Med Outcomes Trust Bull.* **5**: 1, 4.

40 Guyatt GH (1993) The philosophy of health-related quality of life translation. *Qual Life Res.* **2**: 461–5.

41 Leung K and Bond MH (1989) On the empirical iden-
    tification of dimensions for cross-cultural comparisons.
    J Cross-Cult Psychol. **20**: 133–51.

42 Paunonen SV and Ashton MC (1998) The structured assess-
    ment of personality across cultures. *J Cross-Cult Psychol.* **29**:
    150–70.

43 Byrne BM and Campbell TL (1999) Cross-cultural com-
    parisons and the presumption of equivalent measure-
    ment and theoretical structure: a look beneath the surface.
    J Cross-Cult Psychol. **30**: 555–74.

44 Beck AT, Ward CH, Mendelson M, Mock J and Erbaugh J
    (1961) An inventory for measuring depression. *Arch Gen
    Psychiatry.* **4**: 561–71.

45 Nunnally JC (1978) *Psychometric Theory* (2e). McGraw-Hill,
    New York.

46 Deyo RA, Diehr P and Patrick DL (1991) Reproducibility
    and responsiveness of health status measures: statistics and
    strategies for evaluation. *Control Clin Trials.* **12**: 142–58.

47 Ware JE (1987) Standards for validating health measures:
    definition and content. *J Chron Dis.* **40**: 473–80.

48 Aday LA (1989) *Designing and Conducting Health Surveys.*
    Jossey-Bass Publishers, San Francisco, CA.

49 DeVellis RF (1991) *Scale Development: Theory and Applica-
    tion.* Applied Social Research Methods Series. Volume 26.
    Sage Publications, London.

50 Guinot P and Wesnes K (1985) A quality of life scale for the
    elderly: validation by factor analysis. *IRCS Med Sci, Psychol
    Psychiatry.* **13**: 9–10.

51 Bardo JW and Hughey JB (1984) The structure of commun-
    ity satisfaction in a British and an American community.
    J Soc Psychol. **124**: 151–7.

52 Jobe JB and Mingay DJ (1989) Cognitive research im-
    proves questionnaires. *Am J Public Health.* **79**: 1053–5.

53 Patrick DL, Wild DJ, Johnson ES, Wagner TH and
    Martin ML (1994) Cross-cultural validation of quality of
    life measures. In: J Orley and W Kuyken (eds) *Quality of*

Life Assessment: International Perspectives. Springer-Verlag, Berlin.

54 Guyatt GH, Walter S and Norman G (1987) Measuring change over time: assessing the usefulness of evaluative instruments. *J Chron Dis.* **40**: 171–8.

55 Lord FM (1977) A study of item bias, using item characteristic curve theory. In: YH Poortinga (ed.) *Basic Problems in Cross-Cultural Psychology.* Swets and Zeitlinger, Amsterdam.

56 Lord FM (1980) *Applications of Item Response Theory to Practical Testing Problems.* Lawrence Erlbaum, Hillsdale, NJ.

57 Lord FM and Novick MR (1968) *Statistical Theories of Mental Test Scores.* Addison-Wesley, Reading, MA.

58 Streiner DL and Norman GR (1995) *Health Measurement Scales: A Practical Guide to Their Development and Use* (2e). Oxford University Press, Oxford.

59 Linn RL, Levine MV, Hastings CN and Wardrop JL (1981) Item bias in a test of reading comprehension. *Appl Psychol Meas.* **5**: 159–73.

60 Raczek AE, Ware JE, Bjorner JB *et al.* (1998) Comparison of Rasch and summated rating scales constructed from SF-36 physical functioning items in seven countries: results from the IQOLA project. *J Clin Epidemiol.* **51**: 1203–14.

Index

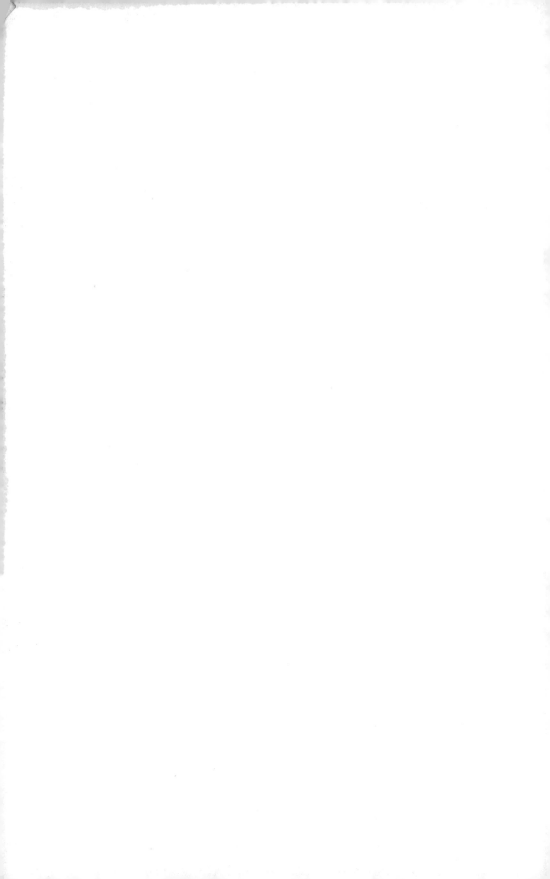